THE NURSE'S CLINICAL SKILLS POCKETBOOK

Sara Miller McCune founded SAGE Publishing in 1965 to support the dissemination of usable knowledge and educate a global community. SAGE publishes more than 1000 journals and over 800 new books each year, spanning a wide range of subject areas. Our growing selection of library products includes archives, data, case studies and video. SAGE remains majority owned by our founder and after her lifetime will become owned by a charitable trust that secures the company's continued independence.

Los Angeles | London | New Delhi | Singapore | Washington DC | Melbourne

Perfect for OSCEs and placements!

THE NURSE'S CLINICAL SKILLS POCKETBOOK

3RD EDITION

EDITED BY
CATHERINE DELVES-YATES

ADVISORY EDITORS:
FIONA EVERETT AND WENDY WRIGHT

Los Angeles | London | New Delhi
Singapore | Washington DC | Melbourne

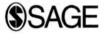

Los Angeles | London | New Delhi
Singapore | Washington DC | Melbourne

SAGE Publications Ltd
1 Oliver's Yard
55 City Road
London EC1Y 1SP

SAGE Publications Inc.
2455 Teller Road
Thousand Oaks, California 91320

SAGE Publications India Pvt Ltd
B 1/I 1 Mohan Cooperative Industrial Area
Mathura Road
New Delhi 110 044

SAGE Publications Asia-Pacific Pte Ltd
3 Church Street
#10-04 Samsung Hub
Singapore 049483

Editor: Alex Clabburn
Assistant editor: Ruth Lilly
Production editor: Martin Fox
Copyeditor: Tom Bedford
Proofreader: Thea Watson
Marketing manager: Ruslana Khatagova
Cover design: Sheila Tong
Typeset by: C&M Digitals (P) Ltd, Chennai, India
Printed in the UK

Library of Congress Control Number: 2022933435

British Library Cataloguing in Publication data

A catalogue record for this book is available from the British Library

ISBN 978-1-5297-9873-9

At SAGE we take sustainability seriously. Most of our products are printed in the UK using responsibly sourced papers and boards. When we print overseas we ensure sustainable papers are used as measured by the PREPS grading system. We undertake an annual audit to monitor our sustainability.

CONTENTS

COMMON ABBREVIATIONS
WENDY WRIGHT AND FIONA EVERETT

Please note you may see the following abbreviations in practice. However, it is best practice to always use the full correct term to prevent mistakes and misunderstandings and to ensure patient safety.

ABG	Arterial Blood Gas
AF	Atrial fibrillation
BP	Blood pressure
C&S/ MC&S	Culture and sensitivity
CCU	Cardiac care unit / Coronary care unit
CO_2	Carbon dioxide
CPR	Cardiopulmonary resuscitation
CSU	Catheter specimen
CXR	Chest x-ray
DOB	Date of birth
DVT	Deep vein thrombosis
ECG	Electrocardiogram
EUA	Examination under anaesthetic
FBC	Full blood count
FBS	Fasting blood sugar
GI	Gastrointestinal
IM	Intramuscular
INR	International normalised ratio
IV	Intravenous
KVO	Keep vein open
MI	Myocardial infarction
MRI	Magnetic resonance imaging
MRSA	Methicillin-resistant Staphylococcus aureus
MSSU/MSU	Midstream specimen of urine
NAD	No abnormalities detected

NIDDM	Non-insulin-dependent diabetes mellitus
NKA	No known allergies
NOK	Next of kin
NSAID	Non-steroidal anti-inflammatory drug
O_2	Oxygen
OT	Occupational therapist
SOB	Short of breath
PR	Per rectum
PRN	Pro re nata (when required)
PUO	Pyrexia of unknown origin
PV	Per vagina
SC	Subcutaneous
SpO_2	Peripheral capillary oxygen saturation
TIA	Transient ischemic attack
TPR	Temperature, pulse, respiration
VS	Vital signs

USEFUL PREFIXES AND SUFFIXES

WENDY WRIGHT AND FIONA EVERETT

A, e.g. asystole	Not, without, less
Ab, Abs, e.g. abduction	From, away from
Ad, e.g. adduction	Toward, in the direction of
Ambi, e.g. ambidextrous	On both sides
Angi(o), e.g. angioplasty	Vessel
Ante, e.g. antecedent	Before
Anti, e.g. antibody	Against, opposing
Arteri(o), e.g. arteriosclerosis	Artery
Arthr(o), e.g. arthroplasty	Joint, articulation
Bi, e.g. bilateral	Twice, double
Brady, e.g. bradycardia	Slow
Bronch, e.g. bronchitis	Bronchus
Cardio, e.g. cardiomyopathy	Heart
Co, e.g. comorbidity	With, together, in association with
Derm/derma/dermato, e.g. dermatology	Skin
Di, e.g. dissect	Separation, taking apart
Dys, e.g. dysphagia	Bad, difficult
Gastro, e.g. gastroenteritis	Stomach, belly
Haemo, e.g. haemotology	Blood
Hyper, e.g. hyperactive	Above, excessive
Hypo, e.g. hypoactive	Below, deficient
Opthalm(o), e.g. ophthalmology	Eye
Pharmaco, e.g. pharmacology	Drug, medicine
Phleb(o), e.g. phlebotomy	Vein
Pneum(o), e.g. pneumothorax	Air, gas, lung, breathing
Poly, e.g. polycystic	Many, multiple
Tachy, e.g. tachycardia	Rapid
Therm(o), e.g. thermostatic	Heat
Thora/thorac(i), e.g. thoracentesis	Chest, thorax
Uni, e.g. unilateral	One, single

INFECTION PREVENTION AND CONTROL

ROSE GALLAGHER

Hand-washing

☑ Before you start

Consider, is it beneficial to inform the patient that you intend to wash your hands? The patient and their relatives or carers may be reassured that you are taking steps to protect them from the transmission of infection via hands.

☑ Essential equipment

Running tepid water, soap, hand towels (preferably disposable, but patients may offer you a clean hand towel in community settings).

☑ Field-specific considerations

Washing your hands is an essential skill within the care of patients from all fields. The principles outlined in this skill will not vary depending on the field.

☑ Care-setting considerations

Facilities for hand-washing will vary considerably between care settings and patients' homes.
  Always be prepared for a lack of running water, soap and clean hand towels.

In community settings, carry your own supply of hand towels or hand wipes to support hand-washing. Always carry hand sanitiser for situations when this is appropriate.

Keep hand sanitisers out of the reach of children or those with impaired mental capacity.

☑ **What to watch out for and action to take**

Do not apply soap directly to dry hands as this can result in sore hands and poor coverage of soap.

Staff with broken skin should cover it with a plaster. Staff unable to perform hand hygiene (because of sore hands) should not be working in clinical environments due to the risks to patients and themselves. Staff suffering from dermatitis and/or sore hands should seek advice from their local occupational health department.

Always use the foot pedal of the bin (if available) – never dispose of hand towels by lifting the lid using your fingers because this will result in recontamination of your hands.

Steps and the reasons for them in hand-washing

Identify the need for hand hygiene to be performed
Undertake an assessment to ascertain whether there is a need for hand-washing to take place.

Turn on taps and select a comfortable temperature
Water that is too hot or too cold can impact on compliance with the hand-washing technique.

Wet hands
Prepare hands to receive soap and facilitate an even covering of soap for the next stage.

Apply soap
Apply one dose of liquid soap to cupped hands.

If bar soap is the only option available, then this may be used, depending on its quality. Community staff may carry small amounts of soap with them in containers.

Rub hands together and evenly distribute soap coverage following steps set out in Appendix 3
Rubbing hands together produces mechanical friction. This results in all areas of the hands coming into contact with soap and transient micro-organisms being lifted from the outer layers of the skin into the soap solution on the hands.

Rinse hands
To remove the transient micro-organisms present in the soap solution from the hands.

Dry hands
Dry the skin of the hands and remove any remaining transient organisms as a result of mechanical friction. Ensure all areas of the hands are dry.

Dispose of hand towels
Dispose of used materials correctly without re-contaminating your hands.

Source: Loveday et al. (2013); NICE (2012a)

Using hand sanitiser

☑ **Before you start**

Consider whether it is appropriate to inform the patient that you are going to use sanitiser on your hands so the patient and their relatives or carers are reassured that you are taking steps to protect them from the transmission of infection via hands.

☑ **Essential equipment**

Hand sanitiser (this may be carried personally, available at the point of care or wall-mounted).

☑ **Field-specific considerations**

Ensuring your hands are free from transient micro-organisms is an essential skill within the care of patients from all fields. The steps outlined in this skill will not vary depending on the field.

☑ Care-setting considerations

Facilities for hand hygiene will vary considerably between care settings and patients' homes.

Always be prepared for a lack of running water, soap and clean hand towels. In community settings, carry your own supply of hand towels or hand wipes to support hand hygiene. Always carry hand sanitiser for situations in which this is appropriate.

Keep hand sanitisers out of the reach of children or those with impaired mental capacity. The ingestion of alcohol hand sanitisers that has resulted in the death of patients has been recorded (HM Coroner, 2017).

☑ What to watch out for and action to take

Any cuts, open wounds or dry skin on hands will sting following the application of hand sanitiser. Staff with broken skin should cover it with a plaster. Staff unable to perform hand hygiene (because of sore hands) should not be working in clinical environments due to the risks to patients and themselves. Staff suffering from dermatitis and/or sore hands should seek advice from their local occupational health department.

Source: RCN (2021)

Steps and the reasons for them in hand hygiene

Identify the requirement for hand hygiene to be performed
Assess whether hand hygiene needs to take place.
   The decision to use sanitiser will depend on being:

- confident that the hand sanitiser will be effective to decontaminate hands. Remember, if a patient has diarrhoea or a gastrointestinal infection such as *C. difficile*, hand sanitiser may not be effective. Wash hands first, if possible, then apply hand sanitiser if needed. Visibly soiled hands should be cleaned with soap and water, if available, or a hand wipe prior to application of sanitiser
- able to access hand sanitiser at the point and time of need.

2 **Apply the hand sanitiser to all surfaces of the hands and rub hands together to support evaporation following steps set out in Appendix 3**

All surfaces of the hands come into contact with the hand sanitiser to ensure transient micro-organisms are destroyed. This six-step technique is more effective than other less standardised techniques (Reilly et al., 2016).

3 **Allow the hand sanitiser sufficient time to dry (evaporate) prior to next patient contact**

The hand sanitiser needs adequate time to be effective and destroy micro-organisms on hands.

When to remove your gloves and why

☑ Before you start

Ensure you have undertaken an assessment to determine if gloves can be retained or should be changed.

☑ Essential equipment

Hand hygiene equipment (soap and water or hand sanitiser).

☑ Field-specific considerations

Mental health – gloves are infrequently used in mental health settings but may be required at times. Indications may include caring for incontinent patients, phlebotomy or dressing wounds. Differences may also be present in practice depending on whether you are working in an inpatient or community setting.

Learning disability nursing – depending on the patients, glove-use need will vary. For those with physical needs, the indications for glove use are the same as for adult general nursing.

Child – indications for glove use in children's settings are the same as for adults, and this includes neonates. Newborn babies may look 'clean' but the same principles and risks apply as with adults.

When there is an indication for hand hygiene
Wearing gloves may afford you some protection but the patient remains vulnerable if you do not consider the risk of transfer of micro-organisms via gloves in the same way as hands.

Whenever an indication for hand hygiene occurs, and gloves are being worn, these should be removed, hand hygiene performed and then clean gloves applied. This is particularly relevant when multiple care activities are undertaken on the same patient.

When glove integrity is breached or suspected
Gloves are not a complete barrier and defects may be present unknown to the wearer. Gloves reduce but do not eliminate risks.

When

a   The actual or potential contact with blood, body fluids or mucous membranes is finished
b   Contact with hazardous drugs or chemicals has finished
c   Contact with a contaminated body site or device (e.g. infected wound, urinary catheter bag) has finished

Once the activity is complete, gloves should be removed, disposed of and hand hygiene performed. This removes potential contamination from the hands of the nurse, protecting both them and the next patient.

Source: NICE (2012a); RCN (2021)

CLINICAL MEASUREMENT

CAROLINE DOBSON AND TREVOR SIMPSON

Fundamental steps for all clinical measurements

☑ What is normal?

Understanding your patient's history and plan of care will ensure you are completing the relevant measurements for your individual patient and it will also help in understanding the individual's normal parameters. Parameters will vary from individual to individual based on many factors such as age, gender, underlying pathology, current medications or treatment or stress. Understanding what is normal is also important so you are able to recognise a deteriorating patient. A systematic approach is utilised in order to undertake a comprehensive assessment of your patient. Therefore, developing the skills and knowledge required to undertake clinical measurements and an A-E assessment is fundamental to all clinical nurses. An A-E assessment facilitates prompt recognition of life-threatening pathology and rapid treatment of deteriorating patients (Japp and Robertson, 2018).

☑ Before you start

Before commencing with any nursing procedure, you need to ensure that you gain informed consent from your patient. In order to do this, you need to establish whether your patient understands what it is they are consenting to by giving them a full explanation of the procedure, including how and why it is being performed. Once an explanation has been given it is important to allow time for any questions they may have, and gauge their understanding by asking them open-ended questions.

☑ Essential equipment

The equipment required will vary depending on the clinical measurement being performed. The most common equipment required is listed below:

- alcohol hand rub or soap and water
- non-sterile gloves
- apron
- fob watch
- waste bag
- measuring equipment, for example manual sphygmomanometer or thermometer.

☑ Field-setting considerations

Anyone over the age of 16 can consent for themselves unless there is evidence to suggest they do not have capacity. However, age, their condition or behaviours should not be considered as a sole deciding factor. If a patient aged under 16 is deemed to understand and have the capacity to consent, they are able to do so (Mental Capacity Act 2005, s.4).

☑ Local policies and procedures

Local policies and procedures may vary depending on where you work, however policies and procedures should always be evidence-based. It is important to familiarise yourself with the local policies and procedures in order to safeguard yourself and your patients. They may require you to undertake a further assessment of competence which will be recorded as part of your continuing professional development.

☑ Care-setting considerations

The guidance for undertaking a procedure in the community may vary from an acute setting due to the staffing and resources available. As the patient's home is not a clinical setting it can be more challenging to provide safe and effective care. Infection prevention policies may differ due to the environment the procedure is taking place in. Risk assessments will be undertaken to determine the level of PPE required to protect both yourselves and your patients (Ward, 2017).

Pre-procedure

Introduce yourself to your patient, and identify you have the correct patient by verifying with the patient and/or checking their wrist band against patient documentation
This promotes patient safety and reduces risk.

Explain the procedure and offer your patient a rationale of why it is required so you can gain informed consent from your patient or carer
If you are unsure whether your patient has capacity seek advice from your practice assessor or supervisor.

Collect required equipment. Ensure it is working correctly and calibrate if required
All equipment will need cleaning in between patient use to prevent the spread of infection. Some equipment, such as blood glucose monitoring strips, will have expiry dates, so ensure all equipment is in date before use. Out of date or uncalibrated equipment may provide incorrect readings which may result in failure to recognise a deteriorating patient.

Wash hands with soap and water using the correct procedure as directed in Infection Prevention and Control
If in a community setting where this is not an option, use alcohol hand gel before the procedure.

Consider the use of PPE such as non-sterile gloves and aprons if appropriate in order to prevent cross contamination

Always maintain your patient's privacy and dignity
They may wish to have the curtains drawn, or doors shut. Offer a chaperone if required to promote holistic patient-centred care, taking into consideration cultural and religious needs.

Ensure they are in a comfortable position before starting the procedure
It may be that you require them to be sat in a chair or laid supine to complete the procedure, for example completing a lying and standing blood pressure. If this is the case explain your rationale to your patient prior to starting.

Post-procedure

1 **Discuss the result of the clinical measurement with your patient**
If they require further information about required interventions seek advice from your practice assessor or supervisor.

2 **Discard any PPE in an appropriate waste disposal container or bag**

3 **Ensure your patient is comfortable and can access help if required**
This may be providing them with a call bell in the acute setting or making sure they can reach the telephone or alert bell if in the community.

4 **Wash hands with soap and water using the correct procedure as directed in Infection Prevention and Control (pp. 1-3)**
If in a community setting where this is not an option, use alcohol hand gel after the procedure.

5 **Document all clinical measurements in your patient's notes**
If there are abnormal findings, escalate to the registered nurse caring for that patient. This is extremely important to ensure there are no delays in recognising and treating deteriorating patients. Failure to do so may result in a worsening of their condition and possibly death (Lister et al., 2020).

Respirations

☑ **What is normal?**

Adults - 12-18 breaths per minute (bpm)

0-1 year - 30-60 bpm

1-3 years - 24-40 bpm

3-5 years - 22-34 bpm

5-15 years - 18-30 bpm

15-17 years - 12-16 bpm

☑ Before you start

When undertaking an assessment of your patient's respiration you need to assess not only the rate of their respirations but also the rhythm and depth. Look at movement of their chest; is it rising and falling equally and bilaterally? Unilateral breathing may indicate your patient has a pneumothorax, which is when the lung has collapsed and is unable to inflate as normal. Is their breathing shallow, indicating they are unable to take a full breath? Shallow breathing could be due to respiratory conditions such as asthma, or other medical conditions such as anxiety. If it is the latter, it may be that you need to provide your patient with some time before measuring their respirations to get an accurate measurement. Talk to them and help them in relieving their anxieties before proceeding. When looking at the chest you can also look for the use of accessory muscles; this can be a good indicator of dyspnoea. Looking at your patient's face can tell a lot about their breathing: note the colour of their skin, look for sign of cyanosis (blue tinge around the lips), this is a sign of hypoxia, or lack of oxygen. You may observe that they are mouth breathing, pursing their lips or flaring their nostrils when breathing. All of these can be signs that they are having difficulty in breathing. Document any findings in your patient's notes.

☑ Essential equipment

You will need a fob watch with a second hand to measure your patient's respirations.

☑ Field setting considerations

Consider your patient and what their normal parameters should be. If you are monitoring respirations on a child, the normal parameters will be higher than an adult. Understand any underlying conditions such as COPD if assessing an adult. The normal parameters will vary due to their condition as well as age.

☑ Care-setting considerations

Many patients are affected by 'white coat' syndrome. This is when anxiety levels increase due to fear of clinical settings or procedures. This is more common if working in an acute setting due to the unfamiliar environment. Discuss any past medical history with them and ensure your patient is relaxed and comfortable before commencing.

Consider steps 1-7 of Clinical measurement guidelines: Pre-procedure (p. 9)
When gaining informed consent observe if your patient is able to speak in full sentences. Inability to do so can indicate a difficulty in breathing.

 Hold your patient's wrist as if checking their pulse
Often when a patient is informed you are counting their breath, they will unconsciously alter their breathing, so acting as if you are checking their pulse whilst counting their respirations will prevent this happening. You can then go on to count their pulse after recording their respirations.

 Count their breaths for one full minute
Do not reduce the time as your patient's breathing may not be regular and insufficient time measuring respiration will not capture this.

 When counting the respirations, observe your patient's chest, looking at the rhythm of the breathing
Rapid, deep breaths are often displayed in patients with diabetic ketoacidosis. It is the body's way of trying to get rid of the excess CO_2 and re-establish the homeostatic balance. This is called Kussmaul breathing and can be noted in both adults and children.

 Observe and document the depth of the breathing. Is it shallow or deep?
Shallow breathing can indicate respiratory distress. You may need to feel the chest if shallow breathing is difficult to visualise. Shallow breathing could be due to fractured ribs or other causes of chest pain. Deep breathing can indicate a neurological injury.

Look to see if the chest is rising and falling equally and bilaterally. Check to see if they are using accessory muscles or signs of recession
Accessory muscles include the sternocleidomastoid, scalene, and trapezius muscles in the neck and shoulders. This may suggest that the intercostal muscles and diaphragm are not working sufficiently to aid pulmonary ventilation (Paton and Elliot, 2017).

7 Whilst recording the breaths per minute also listen for sounds such as stridor, wheeze or gurgling which could indicate obstruction or fluid in the airways

 8 Perform steps 1-5 of Clinical measurement guidelines: Post-procedure (p. 10)

Pulse/heart rate

☑ **What is normal?**

Adult:

- 60-100 beats per minute (bpm)

Child:

- neonate (birth to 28 days) - 100-180 bpm
- infant (28 days to 1 year) - 100-160 bpm
- toddler (1-3 years) - 80-110 bpm
- pre-school child (3-5 years) - 70-110 bpm
- school-aged child (5-15 years) - 65-110 bpm
- adolescent (15-17 years) - 60-90 bpm.

☑ **Before you start**

Your patient should ideally have rested for 10-20 minutes before recording a pulse as exercise or emotional distress may give a false measurement. Consider the site you are going to palpate, for example the radial artery runs closer to the surface of the skin, so it is easier to palpate. It also is easier to access, supporting you in maintaining your patient's dignity whilst undertaking the measurement.

☑ **Essential equipment**

You will need a fob watch with a second hand to measure your patient's respirations, and a stethoscope (if indicated).

☑ Field setting considerations

For neonates and infants, you may need to use a stethoscope to record the apical heart rate. The stethoscope should be placed between the sternum and mid-clavicular line. When checking the pulse in toddlers and pre-school children the brachial artery is often the preferred site to establish the pulse.

☑ Care setting considerations

Consider the environment and document any factors that may affect the patient's pulse, such as stress and time spent resting prior to recording the pulse. If your patient has been running late for an appointment it may be that their pulse will be raised above their normal parameters, so document and re-record after a period of rest.

Pulse/heart rate guidelines

 Consider steps 1-7 of Clinical measurement guidelines: Pre-procedure (p. 9)

 Placing their arm on a cushion will support them whilst you record their pulse

 Place your index and middle fingers over the selected artery at the most appropriate site and apply light pressure until you feel the pulse
Do not use your thumb as you may feel your own pulse, rather than your patient's. You do not need to apply excessive pressure. For the apical heart rate place the stethoscope as discussed above.

 Count the pulse for a full 60 seconds, noting the regularity and strength of the pulse
If the rate is too fast or too slow the cardiac output may be reduced, so document any changes and consider it when assessing other vital signs such as blood pressure.

 You can also use the time to assess your patient's skin condition, for example is it cold, sweaty or clammy to touch

6 Palpation of a radial pulse in an adult can indicate that their systolic blood pressure is above 90mmHg
If you are unable to find a radial pulse, consider palpating the brachial, carotid or femoral arteries

7 Perform steps 1-5 of Clinical measurement guidelines: Post-procedure (p. 10)

Manual blood pressure

☑ **What is normal?**

Age	Systolic	Diastolic
Neonate	60-90 mmHg	20-60 mmHg
Infant	87-105 mmHg	53-66 mmHg
Toddler	95-105 mmHg	53-66 mmHg
Preschool child	95-110 mmHg	56-70 mmHg
School aged child	97-112 mmHg	57-71 mmHg
Adolescent	112-128 mmHg	66-80 mmHg

This table identifies the accepted normal blood pressure values for children and young people, depending upon age.

Low blood pressure (hypotension) is defined as a systolic pressure of below 100 mmHg.

High blood pressure (hypertension) is defined as a systolic pressure of 140 mmHg or higher.

☑ **Before you start**

It is important to assess whether your patient has any of the following conditions/surgeries due to the risk of lymphoedema, further trauma or pain or incorrect readings:

• mastectomy
• arteriovenous fistula
• trauma/surgery

- intravenous infection
- stroke.

☑ Essential equipment

- automatic or manual sphygmomanometer
- stethoscope.

☑ Field setting considerations

Ensure you have the correct size cuff for your patient; they come in varying sizes from neonate to lower limb cuffs. The cuff should be positioned directly onto the skin where possible to gain an accurate recording. Common errors that can affect the reading are positioning the cuff incorrectly, faulty equipment, applying the stethoscope incorrectly and poor positioning of the arm.

☑ Care-setting considerations

Both automatic and manual sphygmomanometers can be used in both acute and community settings, however the use of manual sphygmomanometers is becoming more common within community settings. Automatic sphygmomanometers should be maintained on a regular basis and failure to do so may lead to incorrect BP measurements. Automatic sphygmomanometers should also be avoided in patients with irregular heartbeats due to inaccuracy, so it's important to record a manual pulse prior to starting. It's essential that nurses have the underpinning knowledge and are competent in undertaking manual blood pressures should automated machines not be indicated or available.

Manual blood pressure guidelines

1 **Consider steps 1–7 of Clinical measurement guidelines: Pre-procedure (p. 9)**

2 **Place their arm on a cushion at heart level**
If the arm is lower than the heart it can give a false, high reading. Ask your patient to empty their bladder if possible before proceeding as a full bladder may also cause an increase in blood pressure.

3 Wrap the correct size cuff around the upper arm approximately 2-3 centimetres superior (above) the elbow
If you are unable to use an upper limb you can consider using a lower limb cuff on the thigh.

 4 Ask your patient to remain quiet and still if possible. Movement may affect the reading

 5 Palpate the brachial artery whilst inflating the cuff. Once the pulse can no longer be felt, rapidly inflate the cuff another 20-30 mmHg

 6 Slowly deflate the cuff and when you feel the pulse again, note the reading
This is the estimated systolic pressure. By completing these two steps you are locating the correct position of the brachial artery to apply the stethoscope. Also by estimating the systolic it ensures that when the cuff is re-inflated you are not causing unnecessary discomfort to your patient by overinflating it.

 7 Apply the diaphragm of the stethoscope to the location where the brachial artery was palpated - ensure the stethoscope is switched as per the manufacturer's instructions
Earpieces must be cleaned in between use and inserted facing forwards so the Korotkoff sounds can be heard clearly.

 8 Inflate the cuff 20-30 mmHg above the estimated systolic blood pressure

 9 Slowly release the air in the cuff at a rate of 2-3 mmHg for pulsation. When you hear the first pulsing sound (Korotkoff sounds), note the reading. This is the systolic blood pressure

10 Continue deflating the cuff until you can no longer hear the Korotkoff sounds. When the last sound disappears note the reading. This is the diastolic pressure

11 Fully deflate the cuff and remove from the patient's arm

12 Perform steps 1-5 of Clinical measurement guidelines: Post-procedure (p. 10)

Measuring body temperature

☑ What is normal?

Normal adult range: 36.0–37.0° C.

Normal child range: 36.6–37.7° C.

☑ Essential equipment

The correct thermometer for the site you are using. A number of different types are available: tympanic, oral, temporal and axillary are the sites most often used.

☑ Field-setting considerations

You need to carefully consider which site is the most appropriate to use to measure your patient's temperature. Tympanic thermometers are thought to be the most frequently used, but you would not use this site if a patient had wax, an infection in their ear canal, or if they are younger than 3 months old.

Do not take the temperature of a young child immediately after they have had a bath or been wrapped in blankets, as this is unlikely to give an accurate recording.

☑ Care-setting considerations

Temperature can be measured in any care setting. It is generally non-invasive and is relatively quick to undertake.

Consider the environmental temperature's effect on the patient. It may feel warm to you, but the patient may be immobile and ill, so will need more clothing to keep them warm.

If the patient's temperature is raised, consider removing excess clothing.

☑ What to watch out for and action to take

Assessing your patient's temperature involves observation and feeling, as well as measurement. If the patient's temperature is elevated, they may appear flushed and sweaty. When you are feeling their skin such as by holding their hands, they may feel hot to the touch. Alternatively, if they are cold, they may be shivering, wrapped in clothing or blankets and look pale, and their peripheries may feel cold to the touch.

Temperature guidelines

1 Perform steps 1-7 of Clinical measurement guidelines: Pre-procedure to prepare the patient and yourself to undertake the skill (p. 9)

2 Tympanic: This has become the most commonly used method of measuring temperature in adults, as it is quick, minimally invasive and gives a rapid indication of a change in core temperature as the tympanic membrane is close to the hypothalamus

a Remove the thermometer from the base unit and switch on the device - refer to the instructions as required. (Note: some tympanic thermometers have a setting for use with adults and children)

b Check that the probe tip is clean and intact

c Press the probe tip into the disposable probe cover without touching the cover

d Gently pull the pinna (top of the ear) slightly upward and backwards, so that the ear canal is straightened

e Gently insert the thermometer into the ear canal until it is sealed by the ear canal

f Press the scan button on the thermometer and wait for it to beep

g Gently remove the thermometer from the ear canal and read the temperature displayed on the device

h Dispose of the probe cover by pressing the RELEASE or EJECT button while holding over a clinical waste bag

i Return device to the base unit. (Note: for some devices the base unit will charge the device whilst not in use)

j Accurately record the temperature on the patient documentation

k Avoid using this site if there has been a recent ear infection or there is wax in the ear canals as this can affect readings. Ask patients to remove any hearing aid if there is one in the ear to be used. Use the same ear for readings as anatomical differences can account for a 1°C difference. If the ear canal is not straightened, the reading will not be accurate

3 **Temporal:**

a The temporal artery thermometer is held over the forehead to sense infrared emissions radiating from the skin

b Hold in this position for the specified amount of time (refer to device instructions)

c   Read the temperature displayed

d   Accurately record the temperature on the patient documentation

e   Is quick to use but it has been shown to underestimate temperature

Oral:

a   The oral thermometer probe is commonly connected to a handheld display which also acts as a measuring device. The probe is commonly covered by a disposable plastic sheath. This sheath should be removed and disposed after each reading

b   Digital or disposable thermometers can be used to take oral temperatures

c   For digital oral thermometers, press the probe tip into the disposable probe cover without touching the cover

d   Place the device under the tongue. The patient or the carer may need to hold the probe in position whilst the temperature is being sampled

e   Leave in this position for the specified amount of time (refer to manufacturer's instructions)

f   Read the temperature displayed

g   For digital oral thermometers, dispose of the probe cover by pressing the RELEASE or EJECT button while holding over a clinical waste bag. For disposable thermometers, dispose of the probe cover into a clinical waste bag

h   Accurately record the temperature on the patient documentation

Axillary:

a   Digital or disposable thermometers can be used to take axillary temperatures

b   For digital axillary thermometers, press the probe tip into the disposable probe cover without touching the cover

c   Place the device into the centre of the axilla and place the patient's arm close to their chest wall

d   Leave in this position for the specified amount of time (refer to manufacturer's instructions)

e   Read the temperature displayed

f   For digital axillary thermometers, dispose of the probe cover by pressing the RELEASE or EJECT button while holding over a clinical waste bag. For disposable thermometers, dispose of the probe cover into a clinical waste bag g   Accurately record the temperature on the patient documentation

h   Not as reliable as tympanic measurements for estimating core temperature as there are no main blood vessels around the axilla. Environmental temperature and perspiration can affect accuracy

Ensure that the patient is safe, comfortable and receiving the appropriate care; the results have been documented in the patient's records; the equipment is clean and in working order.

 Perform steps 1-5 of Clinical measurement guidelines: Post-procedure (p. 10)

PAIN ASSESSMENT
ANN KETTYLE

☑ Before you start

If the patient notes are available, review them in order to gain as much information about the patient and their current situation as is possible.

Your assessment should not just focus on the pain itself but also on whether the pain is new, re-occurring or persistent. It is helpful to ask the patient what medication they normally take for the pain and whether they have taken or done anything to alleviate the pain and, more importantly, whether it helped at all.

Gather the appropriate assessment tool and a pen. Make sure that you have something to rest on!

☑ Essential equipment

An appropriate pain assessment tool.

☑ Field-specific considerations

When caring for a patient with a learning disability, it is important to know their level of understanding. You will need to allow time to explain what you are doing. It may be helpful to have the patient's family or carers present.

Patients who have mental health needs may not understand the relevance of what you are doing. Ensure you spend sufficient time explaining this. It may be helpful to have the patient's family or carers present.

Children, younger ones especially, may not understand what you are doing. It is often helpful to have the parents or carers present to assist.

☑ Care-setting considerations

A pain assessment can be undertaken in any care setting.

Always ensure that you have the most appropriate assessment tool available, however you may start with one type to provide appropriate care as soon as possible and then return with a more appropriate assessment tool at a later time or date. For example, in a hospital ward it may be possible to have a variety of assessment tools to hand, however if a patient is being assessed in their own home then you may not have the most appropriate tool.

Comprehensive questions will provide you with an understanding of what pain is being experienced and this will indicate the most appropriate tool to be used on the next visit.

If you feel that the assessment was incomplete, then you should arrange to return as soon as is convenient.

In an acute, hospital-based setting and once a full assessment has been completed, it is easier to provide medication or implement alternative strategies to help alleviate the pain; it is also easier to monitor the effects of the interventions as you see the patient more frequently. Outside of the acute setting, this becomes more difficult as you may only see the patient once a week or even less, however visiting their home will give you the opportunity to observe how they cope with their pain, especially if it is chronic or persistent pain.

Reviewing a patient in their home setting affords you not only the opportunity to establish whether their normal medication is being taken as prescribed, but also whether there is anything else that you can do for them, such as home adaptations.

☑ What to watch out for and action to take

Whilst undertaking a pain assessment, you should also observe for non-verbal cues which may support the patient's answers or provide you with further information.

You should always ask to view the site of the pain and observe for signs of:

- discolouration - any bruises, pale or reddened areas
- open areas or wounds and whether there is any exudate or bleeding - see Skin Integrity (pp. 47-53) for further details relating to the care required
- swelling or inflammation around the site of the pain
- the temperature of the skin around the site of the pain
- any potential concerns - if you are undertaking an initial pain assessment, you also need to consider whether the 'story' around the pain being described is alerting you to a safeguarding concern

- any changes – if you are undertaking a subsequent pain assessment, make sure that you are able to review, compare and discuss any changes in the pain score provided by previous pain assessments with the service user and other healthcare professionals.

☑ **Helpful hints**

- Gloves and aprons must be worn if contact with blood/body fluids/ excreta is anticipated, or the patient is in isolation.
- Hand hygiene must be performed before touching a patient, before clean/aseptic procedures, after body fluid exposure/risk, after touching a patient and after touching a patient's surroundings.
- Waste should be disposed of in a clinical waste bag if it is contaminated with blood/body fluids/excreta.

Undertaking a pain assessment

The first step of any procedure is to introduce yourself to the patient, explain the procedure and gain their consent
Fully informed consent may not always be possible if the patient is a child, has mental health needs or learning disabilities; but even in these circumstances, every effort should be made to explain the procedure in terms that the patient can understand. This is not only respectful of their individual human rights, but also helps to ensure that they will be more accepting of the treatment and that their anxieties are reduced.

Ask the patient whether it is acceptable to them for the assessment to be undertaken where they are
If the patient wishes the assessment to be undertaken in a different area, find an appropriate location.
   Ensure you maintain patient privacy, dignity and comfort at all times.

Identify whether the patient is able to communicate with you or whether they want someone with them, such as an interpreter, a family member or carer, to assist or support the assessment
Ensures that the service user is supported, and their answers are communicated accurately in a timely manner.

Prepare the environment, which includes making sure that the patient is able to see you, that they are as comfortable as possible (you may need to help them get into a comfortable position) and that the conversation is private

Ensure that you position yourself at eye level with the service user without risk to yourself to promote patient comfort and reduce anxiety.

Making sure that the conversation is taking place in a suitable environment will demonstrate respect for the patient and ensure that they feel able to communicate freely.

Throughout the assessment, observe for non-verbal and visual signs of pain, e.g. sweating, grimacing, guarding

Enables you to identify whether the patient is 'holding back' or experiencing pain when they are unable to communicate with you. This is especially important in those with a learning disability or mental health need, where English is a second language, the elderly, the infirm or young children.

Talk to the patient in a gentle and unhurried manner; do not talk too loudly but do make sure that you can be heard

Effective communication is demonstrated, and you are showing respect for the patient's feelings and experience.

Work through the assessment tool and listen to the patient's answers – if you are unclear, ask them to elaborate or explain further

Enables a comprehensive understanding of the patient's feelings and experience and the impact of their pain.

Document answers on the pain assessment tool and in patient notes

Accurate documentation allows for review of the efficacy of interventions and the identification of further interventions.

If a patient identifies that they are in pain or you observe them to be in pain during the assessment, do not complete a full assessment but instead complete a primary assessment:

- Where is the pain?
- How long have they had it?
- Have they had this pain before?

- Have they taken anything for it? If so, did it work at all?
- Are they allergic to anything?
- Do they have any other conditions or take any other medication?
- Other than give medication, is there anything else they would like you to do to help relieve the pain?
- Administer medication and monitor effectiveness.

This primary assessment ensures that the patient is not left in pain for an unacceptable length of time.

Do not delay in obtaining appropriate pain relief - if the patient is in pain now, you need to act efficiently to ensure that they are treated as quickly as possible. Approach a doctor or nurse prescriber immediately to obtain directives for analgesia, or if you are in the patient's own home ask them what they would like to take and whether you can get it for them.

You can return later, when the patient is more comfortable, to complete the assessment.

To ensure appropriate pain control.

On completion of the pain assessment and if there are any previous assessments documented, compare, and discuss with the patient the effect of any interventions previously provided or undertaken by themselves and identify the need for analgesia
Pain assessments should be undertaken whenever the patient's vital signs are recorded or whenever the patient complains of pain. Comparison with previous pain assessments should be undertaken and review of the efficacy of any interventions to identify whether further strategies need to be implemented.

If any changes are noted, report the findings to your practice educator, the doctor or senior nurse in charge and obtain a medication review as soon as possible
This ensures that changes are addressed and that the patient's pain is controlled or that the patient is not on unnecessary medication.

Before leaving the patient, ensure they are in a comfortable position with drinks and call bells available as necessary
Promotes patient comfort and ensures they are well nourished and hydrated. See Assisting People with their Nutritional Needs (pp. 95-123) for more information.

Source: National Institute for Clinical Excellence (2013)

ASEPTIC TECHNIQUE AND SPECIMEN COLLECTION

ROSE GALLAGHER

Principles of asepsis

☑ Field-specific considerations

When caring for a patient with a learning disability, it is important to be mindful of their level of understanding, so that consent and cooperation for the procedure can be gained. You will need to allow time to explain what you are doing and consider whether it will cause discomfort or pain.

Patients who have impaired mental capacity may not understand why you need to undertake an aseptic procedure. They may therefore withhold consent and you may need to refer to local policies on presumed or assumed consent, which will reflect requirements of mental health legislation and best interest.

As younger children may not understand what you wish to do, you may need to modify your approach - it may be helpful to have the parents or carers present to assist.

☑ Care-setting considerations

Aseptic technique can be undertaken in any care setting, although you may need to think carefully about how best to manage the patient and the patient's environment.

☑ What to watch out for and action to take

While undertaking an aseptic procedure, you should also assess:

- the general condition of the patient; specific elements will vary according to the procedure being undertaken (e.g. respiratory rate for care of a chest drain)
- their neurological condition – are they alert and responsive? Are they agitated?
- any signs or complaints of pain or discomfort
- the patient's or relatives'/carers' views – for example, saying that their condition is 'not quite right' or they 'don't feel well'.

The information gained from these observations is additional to any assessment you make relating to, for example, the wound you are dressing and will enable you to fully assess the patient's condition and institute appropriate treatment as necessary, escalating care needs to senior nurses and the medical team.

☑ Helpful hints

- Do I wear gloves and an apron? Gloves and aprons must only be worn if contact with blood/body fluids/excreta is anticipated, or the patient is in source isolation for IPC requirements.
- Hand hygiene must be performed before touching a patient, before clean/ aseptic procedures, after body fluid exposure/risk, after removal of gloves and after touching a patient, or the patient's immediate surroundings.
- Waste should be disposed of into the correct waste stream in line with a risk assessment.

Aseptic technique guidelines

Before commencing any care activity, introduce yourself to the patient, explain the procedure and gain their consent
Fully informed consent may not always be possible if the patient is a child or has impaired mental capacity or learning disabilities, but even in these circumstances, every effort should be made to explain what you are going to do in terms that the patient can understand. This is not only respectful of their individual human rights, but also helps to ensure that they will be more accepting of the treatment and that their anxieties are reduced.

For patients who are unable to provide consent because they are unconscious, refer to local policies.

2 **Assess the procedure and determine its complexity before you start, collecting all equipment that may be needed (and an assistant/chaperone if required)**
Ensures you are fully prepared; also avoids you having to leave the patient or interrupt the procedure.

3 **Consider what is going on around you – do you really need to do an aseptic technique now (even if planned)? Is the patient due to have other investigations that will cause you to rush, e.g. an x-ray?**
Ensures that the environment is conducive to undertaking an aseptic technique – for example, there will be a negative environmental impact if bed-making or cleaning is being undertaken in close proximity to a large wound dressing being undertaken.

4 **Ensure the patient is in a comfortable position where you can access the appropriate area. Ensure the patient has received appropriate analgesia as required**
Promotes patient comfort.

5 **Clear sufficient space within the environment, e.g. around the bed space, chair or treatment area. Ensure the area is private**
Enables clear access for the patient and the nurse to work safely.
Maintains patient privacy, dignity and comfort as required – patients will feel exposed if others can see the care they are receiving.

6 **Transport equipment to the patient appropriately (consider a dressing trolley if available and appropriate)**
Ensures all equipment is to hand.
Maintains cleanliness of equipment and aids transport of all items safely.

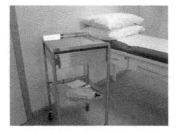

7 **Perform hand hygiene and apply non-sterile gloves only if required**
Wearing apron and gloves is a standard infection prevention practice when dealing with body fluids or patients in isolation if they pose a risk of infection to others.

Ensure your use of PPE is appropriate by considering the individual patient situation and the risk presented. Appropriate hand hygiene will assist in preventing and controlling infection.

Remove and dispose

1 **If present, remove any soiled dressings, 'contaminated' or 'dirty' items and place in appropriate waste bag according to risk assessment**
In preparation for dressing (etc.) change.

Ensure soiled, contaminated or dirty items are disposed of appropriately in the offensive or infectious waste stream depending on risk assessment.

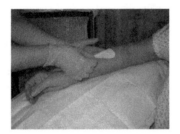

2 **Remove gloves and perform hand hygiene**
Appropriate hand hygiene will assist in preventing and controlling infection.

Create a 'sterile field'

1 **If using a dressing pack, open sterile items and create your 'sterile field' by placing only sterile items within this area**
Creating a sterile field avoids contamination through direct contact with non-sterile items. Remember, your hands are not sterile!

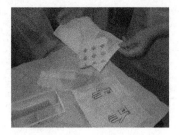

 Apply sterile or non-sterile gloves as required
A risk assessment will determine if sterile or non-sterile gloves are required.

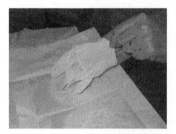 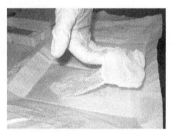

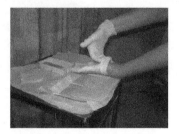

3 **Undertake procedure ensuring:**

- only sterile items come into contact with the susceptible site
- sterile and non-sterile items do not come into contact with each other.

This will prevent and control infection.

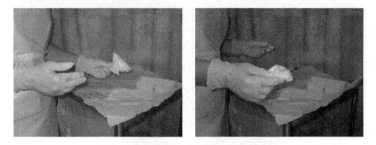

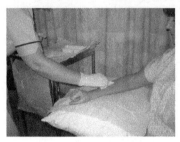

To conclude

After completing the required care, ensure the patient is in a comfortable position, with drinks and call bells available as necessary
Promotes patient comfort and ensures they are well nourished and hydrated.

Dispose of all waste and any single-use equipment, discard PPE (if used) and perform hand hygiene

Clean any equipment used as per the relevant policy every time it is used.
Prevents cross-infection and maintains equipment in working order.

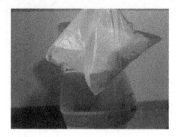

 4 Record the care provided in the patient's record
Maintains patient safety and accurate records.

 5 If any abnormal findings are observed, report to your practice supervisor or a registered nurse immediately
It is vital to report abnormal findings to a registered nurse immediately so they can ensure care is escalated; failure to do so can result in the patient's condition deteriorating and potentially preventable adverse outcomes.

Source: Loveday et al. (2013); NICE (2017); WHO (2009)

Common steps for the collection of all types of specimen

☑ **Essential equipment – depends on the specimen but is likely to include one or more of the following:**

- specimen container, specimen bag and laboratory form
- swabs as appropriate.

☑ **Field-specific considerations**

When collecting a specimen from a patient with a learning disability, it is important to know their level of understanding so that consent and cooperation can be gained. You will need to allow time to explain what you are doing, why you are doing it and whether it will cause discomfort or pain.

Patients who have impaired mental health, including dementia, may not understand why you need to collect a specimen. You may need to refer to local policies on presumed or assumed consent, which will reflect requirements of mental health legislation and best interests.

Younger children may not understand why you need to collect a specimen. You will need to adopt an appropriate approach for consent. It may be helpful to have the parents or carers present to assist.

☑ Care-setting considerations

- Consideration must be given to any equipment needs, e.g. the refrigeration of viral transport media.
- Specimens can be collected in most care settings, however delays in transport to the laboratory may occur outside of hospitals.

☑ Key points to remember

- Ensure there is a clear clinical need for the specimen.
- Explain the rationale to the patient and gain consent.
- The specimen must be obtained without contamination.
- The specimen must be stored appropriately or transferred to a laboratory as soon as possible.
- Check result as soon as available and act on it accordingly.

☑ Helpful hints

- Gloves and aprons must be worn only if contact with blood/body fluids/excreta is anticipated or the patient is in isolation.
- Hand hygiene must be performed before touching a patient, before clean/aseptic procedures, after body fluid exposure/risk, after touching a patient and after touching a patient's surroundings.
- Waste should be disposed of in a waste bag if it is contaminated with blood/body fluids/excreta in line with risk assessment for waste, e.g. offensive or infectious waste.

1 **The first step of any procedure is to introduce yourself to the patient, explain the procedure and gain their consent**

Fully informed consent may not always be possible if the patient is a child or has impaired mental health or learning disabilities, but even in these circumstances, every effort should be made to explain the procedure in terms that the patient can understand. This is not only respectful of their individual human rights, but also helps to ensure that they will be more accepting of the treatment and that their anxieties are reduced.

For patients who are unable to provide consent because they are unconscious, local policies should be referred to.

2 **Ensure that it is an appropriate time to collect the specimen**

The quality of the specimen can be affected by the time of collection and length of time before it reaches the laboratory. To make sure the specimen is of the best quality, ensure that it will reach the laboratory quickly once it has been collected and that it is the best time of day to collect the specimen. For example, it is best to collect a urine sample from the first voided urine in the morning for mycobacterial culture as this will contain the highest concentration of bacteria present.

3 **Gather the equipment required to collect the specimen; ensure this is clean and in working order**

Reduces the chance of inaccurate results.

All lids, containers and specimen bags should be checked to ensure there are no leaks or breaches which could result in spillage during transportation.

Containers used for the collection and transportation of specimens should be CE-marked as this confirms that the container complies with essential requirements – only approved containers should contain specimens for laboratory analysis.

This reduces the chance of infection and helps maintain the quality of the specimen.

4 **Clear sufficient space within the environment where the specimen is to be collected, for example around the bed space or chair**

Enables clear access for the patient and the nurse to safely use the equipment required.

(5) **Standard precautions should be used whenever there is a need to collect specimens**
Wearing an apron and gloves as part of personal protective equipment (PPE) is a standard infection-control procedure when there is contact with body fluids or a patient is in isolation.

Ensure your use of PPE such as gloves and disposable aprons is appropriate by considering the individual patient's situation and the risk presented. Do not use 'just in case'.

(6) **Patients need to be in a private, comfortable and appropriate position and surroundings**
Maintain patient privacy, dignity and comfort as required.

To promote patient comfort and reduce anxiety.

(7) **Complete the appropriate laboratory forms**
The information provided on specimen or laboratory forms is very important. Incorrectly spelled or wrong patient names and identifying information could result in the wrong result being placed in a patient's notes. Alternatively, poorly completed forms could result in specimens being rejected by the laboratory, with significant implications for the patient.

Some organisations use electronically generated specimen request forms and specimen labels to support laboratory tests. Always check local policies for more information.

The laboratory request form must include the following information:

- patient surname and forename (care should be taken to avoid use of nicknames)
- date of birth
- gender
- NHS or hospital number – refer to local policies regarding patient unique identifiers and their use
- location of where specimen obtained (if relevant)
- requesting clinician or consultant in charge
- sample date and time
- name or initial of the person taking the specimen

- clinical information relevant to the specimen - this helps laboratory staff to interpret the clinical significance of specimen results. Examples include symptoms, possible or confirmed diagnosis, any current treatment (e.g. antibiotics) and other pertinent history such as foreign travel.

Some NHS organisations are using barcoding technology to support procedures and trace specimens/equipment used to support patient care. If you are required to use this technology, ensure you have been trained on how to use this before undertaking procedures.

Double-check to ensure the patient is correctly identified - ask the patient (where possible) to state their full name and date of birth. Use patient identifiers (e.g. wristbands) where possible to confirm
Prevents you from taking a specimen from the wrong patient. Never ask 'are you ...?' Always ask the patient to state their name and date of birth.

Some patients may not wear wristbands, e.g. neonates, those living in care homes or those with amputated limbs - check your local policies for alternatives to wristbands.

Ensure specimen is collected in line with local policy
Using an aseptic technique reduces the risk of contaminating the specimen.

Further details relating to taking the following specimens are available within the following:

Sample type	Details
Wound swab	pp. 39-40
Faecal specimen	pp. 41-42
Urine sample	pp. 42-44
Sputum sample	pp. 44-45
Throat swab	pp. 45-46

Specimens for microbiological investigation should ideally be taken before antibiotic therapy is commenced
If the patient is already on antibiotics before a specimen is taken this may have a significant impact on identification of the causative organism (bacteria). The laboratory must be informed

on the laboratory form of all therapy the patient is receiving or has recently received. Where sepsis is suspected, patients should have specimens taken if possible before commencing treatment, however this should not delay the administration of antibiotics.

Specimens for viral investigation can require special transport media

Viruses are generally quite fragile and die easily.

Examples include chickenpox (varicella), chlamydia, influenza, norovirus.

Where specimens are taken directly from lesions, such as vesicles of herpes or chickenpox, then the swab must be placed inside special viral transport media to preserve any viral particles during transport to the laboratory. Viral transport media may require refrigeration and will have an expiry date.

Refer to local policies for more information.

Label container and seal in the specimen bag along with the laboratory request form, in line with local policy

Ensures the specimen and laboratory form are retained together and avoids loss of either during transport.

Specimens should be transported to the laboratory and processed as soon as possible

Once a specimen is obtained, any micro-organisms present have been removed from their 'natural' habitat; therefore in order to preserve micro-organisms, transport to the laboratory should take place as soon as possible. If there is a delay in transportation, some specimens may be refrigerated in a designated refrigerator (do not put in a food fridge) until collection. This is preferable to leaving them at room temperature, which could interfere with the laboratory interpretation of results.

For some specimens, delays of over 48 hours are considered unsatisfactory as the specimen will have deteriorated. Check local policy for further guidelines.

After collecting the specimen, ensure the patient is in a comfortable position, with drinks and call bells available as necessary

Promotes patient comfort and ensures they are well nourished and hydrated.

Discard PPE, any single-use equipment and other used materials as per policy. Clean any equipment used as per the relevant policy and perform hand hygiene
Prevents cross-infection and maintains equipment in working condition.

 Document the specimen collection in the patient's notes
Maintains patient safety and accurate records.

Source: WHO (2009)

Taking a wound swab

Wounds include surgical and traumatic wounds, burns, ulcers, folliculitis and invasive device insertion sites such as an intravenous cannula or wound drain.

☑ Indications for taking the specimen

Wound infection, cellulitis (in the presence of a break in the skin) and/or the presence of pus.

The presence of bacteria in a wound without signs and symptoms of infection reflects colonisation only, and is common in chronic wounds (such as leg ulcers in community settings).

Wound swab guidelines

 Perform steps 1–8 of the Specimen collection guidelines (pp. 35–37)
To prepare the patient and yourself to undertake the task.

 Dip swab in transport media (if present with swab) or moisten with sterile saline
To preserve any bacteria present during transportation to the laboratory.
Moisten swab to avoid dessication of any bacteria present.

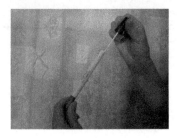

3 **If pus is present, collect pus (via aspiration) or use a moistened swab**
To preserve any bacteria present during transportation to the laboratory.

4 **Take swab from the part of the wound exhibiting symptoms of infection**
This area will produce the best results.

5 **Using an aseptic technique, perform a 'zig-zag' motion while gently rotating the swab between the fingers**
To ensure good contact by the swab with the wound.

6 **Place the wound swab immediately back into the container**
To prevent contamination.

7 **Perform steps for Create a 'sterile field' (pp. 30-32) and steps 9-16 of the Specimen collection guidelines (pp. 37-39)**
To ensure that:

- the patient is safe and comfortable
- the specimen has been correctly collected and documented in the patient's records
- the equipment is clean and in working order.

Source: PHE (2018)

Collecting a faeces specimen

☑ Indications for taking the specimen

Gastro-intestinal infections (bacterial, viral or parasitic) e.g. food poisoning (salmonella, campylobacter, giardia), *C. difficile*, norovirus, shigella, tapeworm.

Ensure the patient actually has diarrhoea in line with local definitions, check with patient if possible and refer to stool chart. If the patient has previously been diagnosed with *C. difficile* infection check with your local infection prevention team and policies for guidance on whether further specimens are required.

Faeces specimen guidelines

Perform steps 1-8 of the Specimen collection guidelines (pp. 35-37) and step 1 of Remove and dispose (p. 30)
To prepare the patient and yourself to undertake the skill.

Negotiate with the patient for them to defecate into a commode or bedpan
To enable a sample to be collected. Support the patient to avoid urinating at the same time. To maintain accurate documentation remember to record specimen collection and bowel motion on stool chart.

Place sample in specimen container carefully avoiding contamination of the outside of the pot
A maximum of 10 g of faeces is suitable for investigation.

Do not overfill the container due to the risk of explosion on opening in the laboratory – natural gases are produced by faecal bacteria so if the specimen is stored in warm conditions a buildup of gas can occur resulting in explosion on opening (with potentially unpleasant results!).

Ensure faeces specimens are transported to the laboratory as soon as possible
Some important organisms, e.g. shigella cysts, do not survive well if specimens are delayed for any length of time.

5 **Perform steps for Create a 'sterile field' (p. 30-32) and steps 9-16 of the Specimen collection guidelines (pp. 37-39)**
To ensure that:

- the patient is safe and comfortable
- the specimen has been correctly collected and documented in the patient's records
- the equipment is clean and in working order.

Source: PHE (2014a)

Collecting a urine specimen

A urine sample includes mid-stream (MSU), clean catch (CCU) and catheter specimen of urine (CSU). Early morning urine (EMU) is required for some tests.

Patients may require support from nursing staff to collect an MSU if they have mobility problems, are elderly or have learning disabilities. Some patients also find the thought of collecting specimens distasteful or undignified and may require support from staff with this. Commercial kits are now available that incorporate a funnel to help patients 'aim' urine into the container and avoid contamination of the outside of the container.

☑ Indications for taking the specimen

Suspected urinary tract infection, other investigation, e.g. legionella antigen test.

EMU for renal tuberculosis or hormonal investigations.

Urine specimen guidelines

1 **Perform steps 1-8 of the Specimen collection guidelines (pp. 35-37) and step 1 of Remove and dispose (p. 30)**
To prepare the patient and yourself to undertake the skill of collecting the required urine specimen.

2 **Advise patient and/or yourself how to collect the specimen (mid stream specimen (MSU), clean catch specimen (CCU) or catheter specimen (CSU))**

CSU

Samples may be obtained from a urethral or supra pubic catheter or as a result of intermittent self-catheterisation.

MSU and CCU

Advice relating to how to collect the specimen will differ according to whether the patient is male or female because of anatomical differences in the urogenital area.

3

Mid-stream specimen (MSU)

The sample should be collected by advising the patient not to urinate immediately into the container but to discard the first few mls of urine.

The first few mls of urine may become contaminated during voiding which could affect the sample quality.

Clean catch specimen (CCU)

All urine is voided into a sterile container and then a portion of this is decanted into a sterile urine specimen container. The laboratory request form must be clear that the urine is a CCU and not an MSU to support laboratory interpretation of results.

Catheter specimen (CSU)

The sample should be removed using a syringe from the dedicated port on the catheter.

The specimen should never be taken from the tap of the catheter bag.

The sampling port should be cleaned with an alcohol wipe if physically clean (if soiled it may be necessary to clean first with detergent and water or detergent wipe).

MSU and CCU

For both male and female patients peri-urethral cleaning is recommended, water is sufficient for this. Separate swabs should be used for each wiping motion and in females the wiping motion should be from front to back to avoid contamination from the anal region.

A CCU is not as good quality as an MSU but is a reasonable alternative where an MSU cannot be obtained.

CSU

Aseptic technique is used to reduce the infection risk.

Historically CSUs were collected using a needle and syringe to access urine via a self-sealing sampling sleeve. This practice is no longer acceptable due to the risk of needle-stick injury.

As necessary place sample in specimen container carefully avoiding contamination of the outside of the pot
10 ml of urine is sufficient for microbiological investigations.

Perform steps for Create a 'sterile field' (p. 30-32) and steps 9-16 of the Specimen collection guidelines (pp. 37-39)
To ensure that:

- the patient is safe and comfortable
- the specimen has been correctly collected and documented in the patients records.

Source: HSE (2013); PHE (2014b)

Collecting a sputum sample

☑ **Indications for taking the specimen**

Upper and lower respiratory tract infections, including pneumonia.
    Micro-organisms normally present in the upper respiratory tract can contaminate the usually sterile lower respiratory tract and cause infection.
    Green sputum does not necessarily mean the patient has an infection!

Sputum sample guidelines

Perform steps 1-8 of the Specimen collection guidelines (pp. 35-37) and step 1 of Remove and dispose (p. 30)
To prepare the patient and yourself to undertake the skill.

The patient is required to expectorate in order to produce a specimen of sputum - saliva is not suitable
Patients who have difficulty coughing or expectorating may need a physiotherapist to help them produce a sample.

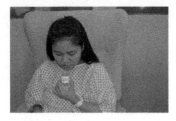

 3 As necessary, place sample in specimen container, carefully avoiding contamination of the outside of the pot
A minimum of 1 ml of sputum is required.

 4 Samples should be sent to the laboratory as soon as possible (sputum may be refrigerated for up to 2-3 hours)
Some bacteria die easily and overgrowth of other bacteria occurs quickly at room temperature, which will produce false results.

 5 Perform steps for Create a 'sterile field' (pp. 30-32) and steps 9-16 of the Specimen collection guidelines (pp. 37-39)
To ensure that:

- the patient is safe and comfortable
- the specimen has been correctly collected and documented in the patient's records
- the equipment is clean and in working order.

Source: PHE (2019)

Taking a throat swab

☑ **Indications for taking the specimen**

To detect a throat infection or carriage of clinically important bacteria, such as MRSA, or occasionally for screening in outbreak or contact situations with, for example, Group A Streptococci, *N. meningitides*.

Throat swab guidelines

Perform steps 1-8 of the Specimen collection guidelines (pp. 35-37) and step 1 of Remove and dispose (p. 30)
To prepare the patient and yourself to undertake the procedure.

Depress the tongue to expose the fauces of the tonsils and gently and quickly rub the swab over the affected or inflamed area
Ensure you have good lighting present to enable you to see into the throat.

The fauces or 'pillars of fauces' are two membranous folds which enclose the tonsils.

Rubbing the swab over the affected area may make the patient gag, obstructing the view of the tonsils.

Avoid contact between the swab and other parts of the mouth (tongue and teeth) as this will contaminate the swab.

Perform steps for Create a 'sterile field' (pp. 30-32) and steps 9-16 of the Specimen collection guidelines (pp. 37-39)
To ensure that:

- the patient is safe and comfortable
- the specimen has been correctly collected and documented in the patient's records
- the equipment is clean and in working order.

Source: PHE (2015)

SKIN INTEGRITY
ALEXANDRA CARLIN

Principles of wound care

☑ What is normal?

Usual patient expectations are for a clean/sterile technique by a competent practitioner, who possesses the necessary skills and knowledge of wound care.

☑ Before you start

Preparation is key: ensure that you have close access to essential equipment.

☑ Essential equipment

- personal protective equipment (PPE) with hand washing facilities
- sterile dressing pack with gauze, sterile field, disposal bag, gallipot (or tray), disposable ruler and gloves
- non-sterile gloves
- wound cleansing solution
- camera for clinical photography
- dressing trolley
- detergent wipes (for trolley)
- swab (in the event of infection)
- appropriate dressings.

☑ **Field-specific considerations**

Younger children may require additional reassurance and support during dressing changes as the process may cause anxiety. With adults, always assume mental capacity unless there is indication otherwise and attempt to involve the patient in the care provided. Carer/family support is encouraged if the person is likely to be distressed during the procedure.

☑ **Care-setting consideration**

Wound care can occur in a range of clinical settings including community, hospital and primary care.

Wound care guidelines

 Introduce yourself to the patient, explain and discuss the procedure with them and gain their consent to proceed
Informed consent should be received prior to all care according to the NMC Code (2018). However, this may not always be possible, for example if the person lacks mental capacity, in which case utilise principles from the Mental Capacity Act 2005.

 Check analgesia requirements, allergy status, religious beliefs and ethical considerations that may affect wound dressing choice
Some dressings may not be suitable due to ethical choices, religion, or allergies, for example an omission of honey in veganism.

 Wash hands with soap and water and put on a disposable plastic apron
You should follow the local infection control procedures in order to prevent cross-infection.

 Clean trolley with a detergent wipe and place equipment required (check integrity of equipment before use).
If a surface is available to you, try to ensure that it is clean and suitable. Ensure that the use by dates of equipment are within range.

5 **Maintain dignity and position patient comfortably so that the wound is easily accessible without unnecessarily exposing the patient**

If you are in a treatment room, use a screen and shut the treatment door. In a patient's home, take them to an appropriate private space and consider closing the curtains.

6 **Clean hands**

To reduce risk of infection.

7 **Open sterile dressing pack using the corners of the paper. Open any other packs (such as dressings) and tip contents gently onto the centre of the sterile field**

There is debate on whether wound care is a sterile or clean procedure. Use your local guidelines. If sterile, try to maintain sterile field and reduce potential contamination.

8 **Clean hands**

Hands may be contaminated when opening dressing packs and handling outer packets.

9 **Using the plastic bag in the pack as a sterile glove, arrange the sterile field**

Pour cleaning solution into gallipot or indented plastic tray. The time the wound is exposed should be kept to a minimum to reduce the risk of contamination.

10 **Attach the plastic bag with used dressing to the side of the trolley below the top shelf on the side next to the patient. Avoid taking the used dressing across the sterile area**

If a trolley is not available, ensure that the bag is not too close to the sterile field (to reduce risk of contamination to the sterile field).

11 **Apply non-sterile gloves, remove, and dispose of any existing dressings. Remove non-sterile gloves**

To reduce risk of cross-infection and prevent contamination of the environment.

12 **Clean hands and apply sterile gloves. To reduce the risk of infection to the wound and contamination of the nurse**

Forceps are no longer recommended for wound care as a gloved hand provides greater sensitivity and is less likely to cause trauma.

13 **If necessary, gently irrigate the wound bed and peri-wound with 0.9% sodium chloride unless another solution is indicated**
A balance must be struck between cleansing the wound to reduce bacterial burden and protecting the wound against physical and chemical trauma to granulation and epithelial tissue from unnecessary wound changes. Tap water might be appropriate depending on the wound. Sterile saline should be used for wound cleaning up to 48 hours after surgery. After that, tap water could be considered. However, if the person is immunosuppressed or risk of infection is high, sterile saline may be more appropriate. If in doubt, seek support from a more senior clinician.

14 **Assess wound healing and obtain wound measurements. If using wound photography, remove gloves, take images, and apply fresh sterile gloves**
Follow your local policies and procedures for wound assessment. If taking clinical photography, consent must be obtained and care taken with the electronic file. Try to upload the file directly into the patient's electronic record. When taking the image, use a sterile ruler beside the wound, with two patient identifiers and the date and time that the image was taken.

15 **Apply appropriate dressing/s and ensure patient comfort**
Dressing selection will vary depending on patient preference, clinician preference, formulary, and the phase of wound healing. Wherever possible, try to achieve dressing selection using a shared decision-making approach.

16 **Dispose of waste in clinical waste bag and any sharps in a sharps bin. Remove gloves, apron, and wash hands**
Follow your local policies and procedures to ensure that the correct disposal processes are adhered to.

17 **Ensure patient comfort and retract curtain (if applicable)**
To maintain dignity and comfort.

18 **Clean hands**
To prevent risk of cross-contamination on the next episode of care.

Source: Lister et al. (2020); National Institute for Care Excellence (NICE, 2019)

Removal of clips/sutures

☑ What is normal?

Usual expectations are for a sterile technique by a competent practitioner with skills and knowledge of wound care. The wound should appear clean and wound edges pulled together with minimal exudate.

☑ Before you start

Explore any resources and documentation provided by the service that inserted the clips or sutures. Establish if the sutures are dissolvable. Ensure that you have close access to essential equipment.

☑ Essential equipment

- PPE with hand washing facilities
- sterile dressing pack containing gauze, sterile field, disposal bag, gallipot (or tray), disposable ruler and gloves
- non-sterile gloves
- wound cleansing solution
- dressing trolley
- detergent wipes (for trolley)
- appropriate dressings
- clip remover or stitch cutter
- swab (in the event of infection)
- sharps bin.

☑ Field-specific considerations

Younger children may require additional reassurance and support during removal of clips/sutures as the process may cause pain and anxiety.

With adults, always assume mental capacity unless there is indication otherwise and attempt to involve the patient in the care provided. Encourage carer/family support if the person is likely to be distressed during the procedure. The patient should remain calm throughout the procedure to prevent injury.

☑ **Care-setting consideration**

Wound care can occur in a range of clinical settings including community, hospital and primary care.

Removal of clips/sutures guidelines

 Introduce yourself to the patient, explain and discuss the procedure with them and gain their consent to proceed

 Perform procedure using aseptic technique
To prevent infection.

 Clean the wound with an appropriate sterile solution such as 0.9% sodium chloride, if required
Crusty scabs and dry skin need to be removed to free the clips/sutures.

 If the incision line is under tension, use a free hand to gently support the skin either side of the surgical incision line
This may reduce skin tension and lessen pain on removal of clip/suture. This is also an opportunity to assess for potential dehiscence.

Clips

 Slide the lower bar of the clip remover with the V-shaped groove under the clip at 90 degrees. Squeeze the handles of the clip remover together to open the clip
If the angle of the clip remover is not correct, the clip will not come out freely.

Repeat until all clips have been removed
Clips should be removed at the earliest point possible to reduce scarring. If there are signs of dehiscence, you may wish to consider removing alternate clips initially and follow up with the patient a few days later to remove the remaining clips.

Sutures

 Lift the knot of the suture with forceps or gloved hand
Plastic forceps will slip against nylon sutures.

 Using a sterile stitch cutter (blade) or scissors, snip the first stitch close to the skin (under the knot). Pull the suture out gently from the knot end
If there are signs of dehiscence, consider removing alternate sutures and then any remaining sutures a few days later.

 Use the tips of the scissors slightly open, or the side of the stitch cutter, to gently press the skin when the suture is being drawn out
Continue until all (if appropriate) sutures are removed. This technique may minimise pain.

 Apply a suitable dressing
To protect the wound from further trauma or contamination and ensure optimum healing.

 Dispose of waste in clinical waste bag and sharps in a sharps bin. Remove gloves and wash hands

 Record the condition of the suture line and surrounding skin
You could consider using the TIME acronym.

Source: Lister et al. (2020); NICE (2019)

SAFE MOVEMENT OF PEOPLE

MICHELLE O'REILLY AND DAVID BEST

Assisted sit to stand with one carer

☑ **Before you start**

- Follow standard infection control procedures.
- Ensure that the patient is sitting in an appropriate style/type/height of chair. If using a wheeled chair apply the brakes.
- Perform a risk assessment. Assess the patient for standing – check their mobility care plan and consult colleagues. The depth of assessment will depend on the handlers' familiarity with the patient and the likelihood that the patient's condition may have changed since the last interaction.
- General observation can be part of the assessment, e.g. looking for signs of good sitting posture. Use your observation skills: is the patient sitting upright in the chair, do they have a weakness on one side or the other?
- To stand with the handler(s), the patient must have a sufficient degree of strength, balance and the ability to understand and follow instructions. An 'on-the-spot' assessment gives an indication of the patient's ability in these spheres.
- Make sure the patient is wearing suitable footwear – close fitting, with non-slip soles. Try to avoid standing the patient in bare feet or with bed socks on. This can cause them to slip.

☑ **Care setting considerations**

- Access to equipment is likely to vary depending on the setting you are working in.
- Remove any obstruction and set up the environment for the transfer to make it easier and safer. Make sure you have enough room to work.

Movement guidelines

 1 Gain the patient's consent and detail what you are both going to do

2 Get the patient to wriggle/shuffle forward in the chair
This makes it easier to stand. If your patient cannot do this, this indicates they have limited core stability/upper body strength and you should use two staff to assist or equipment to stand. If you are not sure stop the transfer and seek help.

3 Ensure the patient's feet are flat on the floor before trying to help them up
If they cannot position at least one foot unaided this should be a cause for concern and will impact on how you move them.

4 Ask the patient not to look down at the floor when standing but to 'lead up with their head, look up with their eyes'

5 The handler then stands at the side of the patient, facing the same direction and angled slightly towards them. The handler's feet should be offset
If your patient has a weakness support that side when going from sit to stand.

6 The handler will then lower their height to take their hold
This should be done in balance, using the principles of safer handling.

7 The handler then takes their hold. With the arm nearest the patient, the handler aims their open hand across the patient's back towards the opposite hip. The handler's forearm is in full contact with the patient's back
Don't grasp clothing or trouser belts.

8 Counter hold – the two most common options used are shoulder or forearm. The shoulder hold means placing your leading arm at the hollow of the clavicle, with fingers pointing upwards
The decision of which counter hold to take should be based on the handler's own risk assessment. Factors such as height of the patient versus the height of the handler(s), any upper limb weakness and whether the patient requires to push on the armrests should be considered. Never lift or use a hold under the armpit.

Encourage the patient to help as much as possible by pushing up on the chair arms or their thighs
Use a simple command such as 'ready and stand' to minimise mixed messages.

On the command to stand, the handler should lead up with their head, and move their feet forward
The most efficient way to do this is to step forward with the outside foot, then follow through with the inside foot. This is a fluid move and brings the handler in line with the patient.

The handler finishes in close to the patient, either beside or slightly behind the patient's hip. The handler's inside foot must remain behind the outside foot to avoid becoming twisted and unbalanced

Make sure to check that the patient is steady on their feet and has any mobility aids they need before releasing your holds

Remember to pass on any changes in the patient's presentation and mobility to other staff in the unit both verbally and in writing

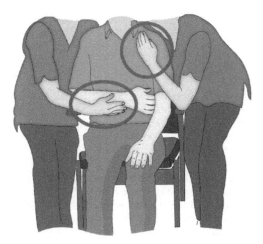

EMERGENCY CARE
SARA MORGAN

Head tilt chin lift

☑ **Before you start**

The safety of the first aider is paramount so ensure that the environment is safe for you to approach. If you suspect the person has a spinal injury move onto a jaw thrust manoeuvre (see p. 59-60).

☑ **Essential equipment**

If in a care setting ensure appropriate PPE is worn.

☑ **Field-specific considerations**

For infants the head should be in a neutral (natural) position.

☑ **Care setting considerations**

The procedure is the same in any care setting.

Head tilt chin lift guidelines

1 If you are able to do so, put on gloves

2 Place one hand on the forehead and three fingers under the chin

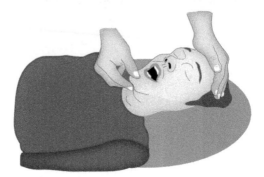

 3 Apply pressure to the chin and lift the chin as you move the head back

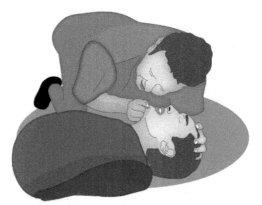

 4 Reassess the airway

5 Has it relieved the problem? If not you may require a definitive airway and expert help

Jaw thrust

☑ **Before you start**

The safety of the first aider is paramount so ensure that the environment is safe for you to approach.

☑ **Essential equipment**

If in a care setting ensure appropriate PPE is worn.

☑ **Field-specific considerations**

There are no field-specific considerations.

☑ **Care setting considerations**

This procedure is the same in any setting.

Jaw thrust guidelines

This is a more complex move to perform; it should be the manoeuvre of choice used in suspected spinal injuries.

 Place your fingers under the angle of the jaw

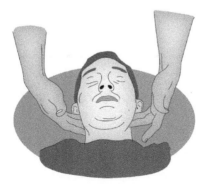

2 Place thumbs on the mandible

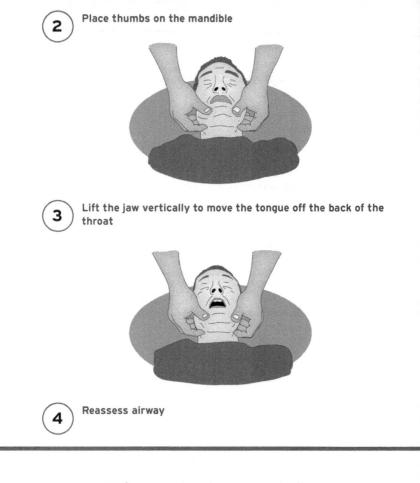

3 Lift the jaw vertically to move the tongue off the back of the throat

4 Reassess airway

Using an oropharyngeal airway

☑ **Before you start**

Assess the person for any signs of facial trauma.

☑ Essential equipment

Appropriate PPE.
   Oropharyngeal airway.

☑ Field-specific considerations

In children under 8 years of age the airway should be inserted concave side down using a tongue depressor.

☑ Care-setting considerations

This procedure is the same in any care setting.

Oropharyngeal airway guidelines

 Measure the airway from the angle of the jaw to the corner of the mouth

 Insert the airway upside down (concave side up) and position to the junction of the hard and soft palate

3 Rotate the airway 180 degrees, so the airway lies in the oropharynx (Resuscitation Council UK, 2021)

Recovery position

☑ Before you start

Risk assess the environment to make sure it is safe to approach the person.
   Ensure that you maintain principles of good manual handling.

☑ Essential equipment

Appropriate PPE.

☑ Field-specific considerations

If the person is known to have learning difficulties or cognitive impairment it may not be possible to ascertain their level of understanding. If the person is not known to the first aider, a relative or carer may be able to give more information.

☑ Care-setting considerations

This procedure can be undertaken in any care setting.

Recovery position guidelines

1 Place the arm closest to you at a right angle

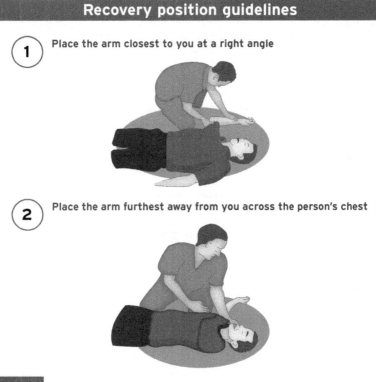

2 Place the arm furthest away from you across the person's chest

3 Bend the leg furthest away from you at 90 degrees

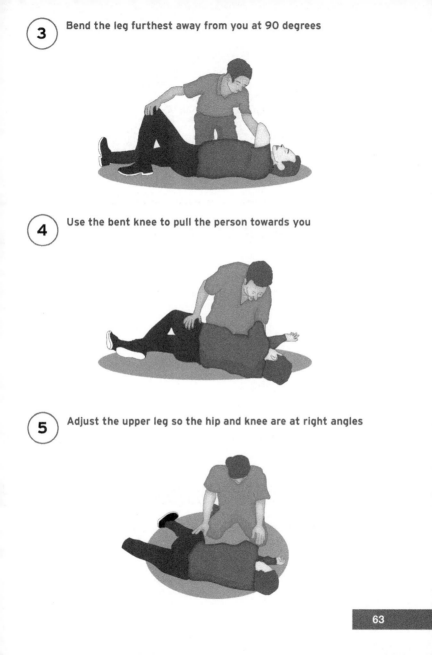

4 Use the bent knee to pull the person towards you

5 Adjust the upper leg so the hip and knee are at right angles

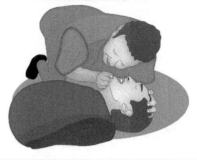

6 Perform a head tilt chin lift to protect the airway

Paediatric life support

☑ What is normal?

Only ever perform this skill upon a collapsed, unresponsive child or infant with no signs of life.

☑ Before you start

Remember to assess the safety of the environment before you start.

☑ Care-setting considerations

This can be undertaken in any care setting.
  It is also important to remember that some form of resuscitation is better than doing nothing.

Paediatric life support guidelines

 1 Check if the child is responsive; in infants, tickling the feet usually elicits a response. Do not shake children

 2 If there is no response, shout for help

(3) **To open a child's airway use the head tilt chin lift manoeuvre; in infants keep the head in a neutral position.**
As children's airways are delicate be careful not to push on the soft tissue under the chin as this may block the airway (Resuscitation Council UK, 2021)

(4) **If there are no visible chest movements, you will need to administer five rescue breaths**
In babies and infants you can make a seal with your mouth around both their lips and nose in order to deliver the rescue breaths.

(5) **If there are no signs of life you will need to start chest compressions. In children under 1 year old the tips of two fingers should be used in the middle of the chest. In children over 1 year use the heel of one hand placed one finger width above the xiphisternum. Compressions should be at a ratio of 15 compressions to two rescue breaths**
If you are a lone rescuer and no help is available you should undertake one minute of resuscitation before calling for help. With younger children it may be possible to carry the child whilst gaining help.

If a defibrillator is available, although a primary cardiac arrest is rare, you should still attach it to the child.

Dislodging an obstruction to the airway

☑ What is normal?

Distressed person, may or may not be coughing.

☑ Before you start

Perform a risk assessment and ensure the environment is safe before you approach the person.

☑ Field-specific considerations

In infants remember to use back slaps and chest thrusts.

☑ Care-setting considerations

Can be managed in any care setting.

Dislodging an obstruction to the airway guidelines

 If the person is conscious administer five back blows; if this does not clear the obstruction you must then deliver up to five abdominal thrusts (not for children or infants)
These steps should be carried out whilst the person is conscious and until the obstruction is dislodged

 In order to perform abdominal thrusts you should stand behind the adult, place your arms around them, put a clenched fist of one hand in the centre of the chest, grasp with the other hand and push upwards (Simpson, 2016)

 If the person is unconscious either call 999 or (if in hospital) the cardiac arrest team immediately
Chest thrusts cause greater airway pressures than abdominal thrusts; in the unconscious person, CPR mimics this movement and should be commenced immediately (Kinoshita et al., 2015).

In children

 If the child has an effective cough encourage them to clear the obstruction. If the cough is ineffective call 999 or (if in hospital) the cardiac arrest team immediately

 In small children and infants place the child in a head down position, supporting the head, and deliver five back blows

 In older children follow the same actions as for adults

 For infants under 1 year, you will need to deliver chest thrusts, one finger breadth above the xiphisternum, at a rate of 20 chest thrusts per minute

(Verma, 2011)

MEDICINES ADMINISTRATION

CAROL HALL, UPDATED BY CHRISTINA ROULSTON

Administering medication (oral or topical route)

☑ **Essential equipment**

- drug to be administered
- medication pots (or suitable vessel) to take the drug to the patient in
- jug of water and clean glasses
- Medicine Administration Record.

☑ **Field-specific considerations**

When caring for patients, it is important to remember that many have needs which cross the boundaries of the fields of nursing, so consider all of this information as potentially relevant to the patients you may care for.

It is important at all times to empower all patients with respect to medicine administration.

Learning disability – ensure that the patient and their main carers, as appropriate, are informed about their medicine and about how it assists them. To do this you need to undertake an assessment of the individual's capability. Some people with a learning disability will be able to manage their own medications, while others may need varying amounts of support. The use of preloaded and timed pill boxes may be useful in some cases to establish a regular routine and to ensure that your patient takes the correct medicine. Medication Administration Records which include a photograph of the individual are frequently used in community settings as they provide a safe method of identifying an individual (as identity bands are unlikely to be worn). Another method can be the use of two identifiers (for instance, name and date of birth as well as photo or ID band).

Mental health – the use of physical and psychological supportive techniques and a good understanding of how your patient feels about their medications will assist you in appreciating the extent to which the monitoring of medications and support is required. Remember that some patients will be receiving treatment under the Mental Health Act, so may not wish to comply with this. It is also important to consider different models of health belief and self-care in establishing the best care possible for your patient. The therapeutic relationship you have with your patient will influence the information they share in respect of their drug treatment. Remember that other forms of treatment, such as psychotherapy, counselling or cognitive behavioural therapies, may be in effect simultaneously with medication. For some patients with mental health problems, including those who are severely depressed or with suicidal tendencies, when administering medicines you must ensure any medicines given to your patient have been taken. It is important to be aware that medicines may be hidden in the mouth and then secretly stockpiled.

Child – encourage, assist and educate children of all ages, as well as their parents or carers, to be involved in the administration of medicines. This will enable you to determine the capabilities the child may have, their likely behaviour and their understanding of the situation. Ensure you tailor your communication skills to reflect the needs of different age groups. An awareness of pharmacology and calculation skills to work out patient-specific drug doses is necessary in all fields, but since many drug dosages are determined by a child's weight in kilograms it is essential in this field of nursing. It is important that any medication administration is always undertaken away from 'safe' areas, such as the playroom or bedside, especially if the medicine administration is unpleasant. For neonates or in specialised circumstances, you may also need to learn to calculate very small doses using micrograms.

Adult – in adult nursing, all of the above might apply, and your role involves assessing a diverse range of individuals who need your care. While most adults will be able to actively participate in their treatment, you will certainly encounter patients with dementia and those who are confused.

☑ Care-setting considerations

It is possible for medications to be administered orally or topically in all care settings.

☑ What to watch out for and action to take

Monitor the effectiveness of the treatment by pre- and post-administration observations. For example, has the patient's temperature reduced? Is the patient still in pain, or feeling nauseous, following the administration of medication?

Ensure you are aware of the therapeutic application of the medicine to be administered, its normal dosage, side-effects, precautions and contraindications before you administer it. Ensure you refer to an up-to-date version of the British National Formulary (BNF) to ascertain this information before administering any medicines with which you are unfamiliar.

Monitor for any reactions to the medication, report any concerns to your practice supervisor or a registered nurse and ensure they report this to the person prescribing the drug without delay. All drug reactions need to be treated appropriately as soon as they become apparent.

Contact the person prescribing the drug if an assessment of the patient indicates that the medicine is no longer suitable or the patient declines to take it.

☑ Helpful hints

- Gloves and aprons must be worn if contact with blood/body fluids/excreta is anticipated or the patient is in isolation.
- Gloves should be worn if contact with the medication is potentially harmful to the nurse – for example, in the case of topical steroid preparations.
- Hand hygiene must be performed before touching a patient, before clean/aseptic procedures, after body fluid exposure/risk, after touching a patient and after touching a patient's surroundings.
- Waste should be disposed of in a clinical waste bag if it is contaminated with blood/body fluids/excreta.

To aid you to administer oral medications safely, always follow the top tips below.

Top tips for administering oral medications

- Check the prescription chart and the BNF for any special instructions relating to how to administer medications, such as:
  - administer with food, before food or after food
  - any possible interactions with other medications, substances such as herbal medicines or grapefruit juice
  - 'slow-release' tablets must be swallowed whole to allow the medication to be released gradually.

- Do not crush coated tablets as in doing this you are making their use unlicensed.
- Do not break tablets that are unscored as you are likely to be giving an inaccurate dose.
- If medication is to be administered via a nasogastric (NG) or percutaneous endoscopic gastrostomy (PEG) tube, ask the pharmacist to dispense a suspension which will not block the tube.
- If a medication is in liquid form, shake the bottle before you pour it out to ensure it is evenly concentrated.
- When using a medicine pot to measure a liquid, place it on a flat surface and ensure you are at eye level to it in order to read the graduations accurately.
- As well as being ingested via an oral route, tablets may be administered via the:
  - sublingual route, which means they are placed under the tongue
  - buccal route, which means they are placed between the cheek and the upper gum.
- Liquids can be administered via an NG or PEG tube.

(Hall, 2018)

Medicine administration guidelines

Ensuring safe and effective storage and administration of medication to patients

Introduce yourself to the patient, explain the procedure and gain their consent
Adapt communication style to meet the needs of the individual patient and their family or carers.

Patients should be involved as desired in decisions relating to their medicines. Fully informed consent may be difficult if the patient is a child or has severe mental health issues or learning disabilities, but every effort should be made to explain the procedure in a way the patient can understand. This is respectful of individual human rights, supports informed participation and reduces anxiety. For patients unable to provide consent because they are unconscious, advice should be sought from your practice supervisor or another qualified nurse.

Gather required equipment
Ensure cleanliness.
Reduces risk of cross-infection and maintains patient and nurse safety.

Identify an appropriate place to prepare medications, away from interruptions and distractions
Clear sufficient space within the environment where the drug is administered.
Ensures patient safety, as interruption is associated with medication error.
Enables clear access for the patient and the nurse to safely administer the medication.

Wash your hands with soap and water before you start administering medication. Ensure your use of personal protective equipment (PPE) such as gloves and disposable aprons is appropriate by considering the individual patient situation and the risk presented
Wearing an apron and gloves as part of PPE is standard infection control procedure when dealing with body fluids or patients in isolation. When administering medications, you may need to wear gloves to protect yourself from exposure to the drug (such as when applying topical skin preparations).

Follow local policy for the administration of medicines. This may mean you must observe rather than participate in administration directly yourself. As a nursing student, you must ensure you are supervised by a registered nurse when administering medication
To ensure patient safety and support your learning.
To meet local policy guidance requirements which ensure employees and students are fully insured for the care that they give.

Before you give any medication, you will need to complete a full assessment of your patient's medication needs. This involves:

a   Checking the patient's care plan for specific requirements
b   Checking the Medicine Administration Record to determine the correct medicine to be given to the correct patient, taking account of all eight rights of medicine administration.

To ensure patient safety.

You need to be aware of the patient's plan of care to ensure no changes have been made and that the medication administration remains appropriate.

To ensure the drug is administered accurately and safely.

Medicines must be given in a timely manner in order to ensure optimum benefits from treatments.

It is dangerous to administer a medication which is not specifically licensed for a particular route.

(7) If a number of medicines need to be given at the same time, prioritise which one to administer first

Some medicines require specific conditions for best effect.

If the medications are to be administered orally, it may be possible for the patient to take them simultaneously provided they do not interact with one another. If medication is required via different routes (e.g. injection and oral), then this will need to be managed to enable optimum treatment. Seek advice from the pharmacist.

(8) Decide if there is reason not to administer the medicine at this time and record and report accordingly

If there has been a change in the patient's condition, a medication may no longer be appropriate, or the patient may be unable to take it. If a patient is 'nil by mouth', check with the drug prescriber whether any of their oral drugs still need to be given (for example, cardiac drugs), possibly by a different route.

(9) Locate medicine to be administered, ensuring it is:

a   In date
b   The correct formulation for the route to be given and appropriate for your patient's preferences
c   The correct dose strength for the prescription
d   The correct medicine according to the prescription.

The quality of an out-of-date medicine may have deteriorated

To prevent error and ensure the best possible outcome in terms of patient care

To ensure safe practice, as medicines are available in different strengths

You must check that the prescription and the label on the medicine are both clearly written and are the same to ensure patient safety

10 **If your patient is a child or the drug dose is calculated according to the patient's weight, check that the prescribed dose is correct for the patient's current weight or BMI**

To ensure patient safety, the dose must be checked using accurate patient weight. Some adult drugs are prescribed according to patient weight to ensure accuracy of treatment. Patient weights can change considerably through the illness process.

Children's medicines are calculated on the basis of milligrams per kilogram per day. Some specialised areas use BMI and surface area for drug doses. A calculator can be found on the BNF website.

11 **Calculate the amount of medicine to administer and measure the required amount accurately**

An accurate amount of medication must be given to the patient.

Medicine must always be measured accurately using appropriate equipment. For example, measuring a dose of 5 ml using a 50 ml medicine pot makes accuracy difficult. The difference of even a few ml can cause problems. Always use the smallest appropriate measuring device.

12 **Ensure medication is placed in an appropriate receptacle for administration to the patient**

To make taking the medicine as easy as possible for the patient.

13 **Medication which is not needed must be returned to its place of secure storage or disposed of in accordance with local policy and legal requirements**

Safe disposal of medicine is important to keep patients, families, carers and staff safe from unwanted effects. Controlled medicines and highly toxic materials will have specific handling and disposal guidelines.

14 **Complete final checks, which always include patient identity and allergies, but may also include specific checks for individual drugs. Provide patients with necessary information regarding their medication, using an appropriate means of communication to aid explanation**

To ensure patient safety:

a   Be certain of the identity of the patient to whom the medicine is to be administered

b   Check that the patient is not allergic to the medicine before administering it

c   Before administering some drugs, cardiac ones for example,
     it is necessary to check that the patient's heart rate or blood
     pressure is within acceptable parameters.

Patients and carers must be aware of the main features of
the medicines given and how to manage them effectively and
concordantly. They need to know what to do if the medicine is
taken inappropriately and the implications of missing doses.

**Ensure your patient is fully prepared for the administration
of the medication and is in an appropriate position. Provide
protective clothing or tissues if needed, or a drink, etc. An
infant may need to be held securely**
Patients should be in a position which ensures both comfort and
safety.

    Protective clothing can maintain dignity through avoiding spills.

**Ensure medication is administered in accordance with the
prescription, local policy and patient preferences (see steps for
Administering medication (oral or topical route), p. 67). If given
orally, ensure medication has been swallowed**
To ensure patient safety and involvement and that the medication
is received as prescribed.

Recording administration and outcome

**Record that the medicine has been administered on the
Medication Administration Record to ensure a legal record of
the medicine administered**
You must make a clear, accurate and immediate record of all
medicine administered, or any intentionally withheld or refused
by the patient. You must ensure your signature is valid and is
clear and legible. If local policy has allowed you to administer
the medication, ensure the registered nurse supervising you
countersigns your signature.

    Evaluation of the impact and effectiveness of the medication
and assessment of any untoward events.

**Document relevant information on the patient's observation
chart and/or in the patient's notes as necessary**
Monitor the effectiveness of the medication and any reactions,
reporting these to a registered nurse and the medication
prescriber and instigating treatment as appropriate.

Maintains patient safety and accurate records. Failing to complete documents may mean a patient could receive the medication on more than one occasion.

Ensure you are fully aware of the therapeutic uses of the medicine to be administered, its normal dosage, side-effects, precautions and contraindications.

Adverse reactions to medications can range from discomforting to life-threatening. By administering a medicine, you undertake to ensure that you are aware of any possible reactions and know what to do in response.

Ensure you advise patients of any signs to watch out for and identify how they can inform you.

(19) After the medication administration has been completed, ensure the patient is in a comfortable position, with drinks and call bells available as necessary
Promotes patient comfort and ensures they are well nourished and hydrated.

(20) Discard PPE, any single-use equipment and other used materials as per policy. Clean any equipment used as per the relevant policy every time it is used and perform hand hygiene
Prevents cross-infection and maintains equipment in working condition.

Source: BNF (2021); NPC (n.d.); Westbrook et al. (2010); WHO (2009)

Administering a subcutaneous injection

☑ Essential equipment

Drug to be administered, either in a prefilled syringe with a nondetachable needle or in an ampoule, sterile swab (to open ampoule), blunt fill needle (to draw up drug if not using a prefilled syringe, with a filter if drawing up from a glass ampoule), safety needle (to give drug if not using a prefilled syringe; choice depends upon patient and drug to be given), appropriately sized syringe, injection tray (or similar), gloves, sharps bin, spot plaster (or similar) to cover injection site.

Medicine Administration Record.

☑ Field specific considerations

Refer to Administering medication (pp. 67-75).

It is not uncommon for both adults and children to be very worried about having an injection. Make sure you take time to relax the patient as much as is possible and answer any questions they have. The patient may wish to have another person they trust present for the procedure (or it might be necessary to have the assistance of another member of the healthcare team or a play specialist), to hold the patient's hand and distract their attention by, for example, talking, story-telling, singing etc. (Local anaesthetic creams are frequently used prior to subcutaneous administration of medicines in children.)

☑ Care setting considerations

It is possible for subcutaneous injections to be administered in all care settings.

☑ What to watch out for and action to take

Refer to Administering medication (pp. 67-75).

- Subcutaneous injections are given into the fatty layer of tissue just under the skin. As blood flow to fatty tissue is relatively poor, any medication given by this route will be absorbed slowly, sometimes taking up to 24 hours.
- Never give a subcutaneous injection into skin that is burned, hardened, inflamed, swollen or damaged by a previous injection.
- There are a number of sites where subcutaneous injections are frequently given. The site chosen will depend upon the volume of medication to be given and how thick it is, plus the amount of subcutaneous tissue the patient has at the injection site. The site to be used should be decided upon after consideration of these factors and take into account the patient's preference. When a patient is receiving regular subcutaneous injections it is important to rotate the site, to prevent scarring and hardening of the tissue.
- Do not give a subcutaneous injection within 5 cm of the navel or any scar tissue.
- It is not necessary to decontaminate socially clean skin with an alcohol wipe prior to administering a subcutaneous injection as alcohol causes the skin to harden, which will alter absorption of the medication when the site is next used.

- If the skin is visibly soiled decontamination using an alcohol wipe is appropriate.
- When administering an injection ensure that you always adhere to all of the relevant policies outlined by the healthcare provider and your educational institution.

☑ Helpful hints

- Gloves and aprons must be worn if contact with blood/body fluids/ excreta is anticipated or the patient is in isolation.
- Gloves must be worn for all invasive procedures and all activities carrying a risk of exposure to blood, body fluids or to sharp or contaminated instruments.
- Gloves should be worn if contact with the medication is potentially harmful to the nurse.
- Hand hygiene must be performed before touching a patient, before clean/aseptic procedures, after body fluid exposure/risk, after touching a patient and after touching a patient's surroundings.
- Waste should be disposed of in a clinical waste bag if it is contaminated with blood/body fluids/excreta.

Administering a subcutaneous injection guidelines

Ensuring safe and effective storage and administration of medication to patients

Remember that as a nursing student you need to be supervised at all times by a registered nurse when administering medication
To ensure patient safety and support your learning.

Identify an appropriate place to check the patient's medication, away from interruptions and distractions
To ensure patient safety as interruption is associated with medication error.

Before you give any medication you will need to complete an assessment of your patient's medication needs. This involves:

a   Checking the patient's care plan for specific requirements

To ensure patient safety:

- you need to be aware of the patient's plan of care to ensure no changes have been made and that the medication administration remains appropriate
- to ensure the drug is administered accurately and safely.

b   Checking the Medicine Administration Record to determine the correct medicine to be given by subcutaneous injection to the correct patient, taking account of all eight rights of medicine administration

- Medicines must be given in a timely manner in order to ensure optimum benefits from treatments.
- It is dangerous to administer a medication which does not have a specific licence for a particular route.

Decide if there is any reason not to administer the subcutaneous injection at this time and record and report accordingly
If there has been a change in the patient's condition a medication may no longer be appropriate.

Ensure the drug to be administered by subcutaneous injection is:

a   In date
b   In the correct dose for the prescription
c   The correct medicine according to the prescription.

The quality of an out of date medicine may have deteriorated.
    To prevent error and ensure the best possible outcome in terms of patient care.
    To ensure safe practice as medicines are available in different strengths.
    You must check that the prescription is clearly written and the medication is the same to ensure patient safety.
    You must never give a medicine without being certain that the dosage (relating to the patient's weight where appropriate), the method of administration, the route and the timing are all correct.

If your patient is a child or the drug dose has been calculated taking account of the patient's weight, check that the prescribed dose is correct for the patient's current weight or BMI
Children's medicines are calculated on the basis of milligrams per kilogram per day. Some adult drugs are prescribed at a dose which

takes account of the patient's weight. To ensure patient safety the dose must be checked, using an accurate patient weight.

Some specialised children's areas use BMI and surface area for drug doses. A calculator for this can be found at the BNF for children online at https://bnf.nice.org.uk

Injections should be prepared in a clean area using an aseptic non-touch technique
To reduce the risk of infection.

If using a prefilled syringe this step is not required as the drug is already in the syringe!
If drawing up the drug:

a   Attach a blunt fill needle to the syringe. Make sure you use one with a filter if you are drawing a drug up from a glass ampoule.
b   If the drug is in a glass ampoule, flick it to remove any medication from the top.
c   Cover the top of the ampoule with a sterile swab and snap it off along the score lines at the neck.
d   Check that there are no particles of glass in the medication; if there are, use a new ampoule.
e   Draw the drug up into the syringe.
f   Holding the syringe upright, with the needle at the top, tap the side of the syringe.
g   Expel the air and any excess medication.
h   Remove the fill needle and dispose of it in the sharps bin.
i   Attach the safety needle to be used to administer the medication using a non-touch technique.

Either 27G or 31G safety needles are frequently chosen to administer medication subcutaneously
a   To reduce the risk of glass particles being drawn up with the medication.
b   To ensure all medication is drawn up.
c   To remove the medication safely from the ampoule.
d   To ensure the medication given to the patient does not contain glass.
e   To encourage any air bubbles to rise so they can be expelled.
f   To leave the correct dose in the syringe.
g   To ensure safety.
h   The choice of needle depends upon the patient's size and the viscosity of the medication.

Place the syringe containing the medication on an injection tray with a spot plaster and take it to the patient with the Medicines Administration Record. Ensure a sharps bin is to hand

To safely dispose of the syringe once the medication has been administered.

Every effort should be made to explain the procedure in terms that the patient can understand. This is not only respectful of their individual human rights, but also helps to ensure that they will be more accepting of the treatment and that their anxieties are reduced.

 Introduce yourself to the patient, explain the procedure and gain their consent

Ensure that you adapt your communication style to meet the needs of the individual patient and their family or carers as relevant.

All patients should be offered the opportunity to be involved in decisions relating to their medicines at the level they wish.

For patients who are unable to provide consent because they are unconscious, advice should be sought.

 Clear sufficient space within the environment where the drug will be administered. Place the injection tray containing the syringe in a safe place where you can see it at all times

Enables clear access for the patient and the nurse to safely administer the medication.

To ensure patient safety whilst you complete the next step.

Complete the final checks, which always include patient identity and allergies but may also include specific checks for individual drugs. Provide patient with necessary information regarding their medication, using appropriate means of communication to aid explanation

To ensure patient safety you must:

a   Be certain of the identity of the patient to whom the medicine is to be administered

b   Check that the patient is not allergic to the medicine before administering it

c   Before administering some drugs, cardiac ones for example, it is necessary to check that the patient's heart rate or blood pressure is not too low.

Patients, their families and carers need to be aware of the main features of the medicines given and how to manage them effectively and concordantly. They need to know what to do if the medicine is taken inappropriately and the implications of not taking it.

Decide which injection site is going to be used

Ensure your patient is fully prepared for the administration of the subcutaneous injection and is in an appropriate position. An infant may need to be held securely.

Offer the patient the opportunity to be involved in the decision of choice of site as appropriate.

Patients should be in a position which ensures both comfort and safety.

Ask and/or assist the patient to remove their clothing as is necessary to expose the injection site

Ensure you maintain the patient's dignity and privacy.

Perform hand hygiene and put on gloves

Remove the cover from the needle of the syringe, taking care not to contaminate it.

To reduce the chance of infection gloves must be worn for all invasive procedures and all activities carrying a risk of exposure to blood, body fluids or to sharp or contaminated instruments.

To ensure the needle is not contaminated.

Hold the syringe like a pencil in the hand you write with. Ensure the needle is pointing towards the patient. Gently pinch the patient's skin at the chosen site between the thumb and first finger with your other hand. The fold of pinched skin should be approximately twice as long as the needle

Pinching up the skin between your thumb and first finger ensures that the subcutaneous tissue is separated from the muscle below. If the skin is not pinched up, it could result in administering the medication into the muscle rather than the subcutaneous tissue.

Quickly insert the needle all the way into the fold of skin at an angle of 90 degrees, unless a different angle is recommended by the manufacturer. Do not push the needle into the skin slowly or stab the needle into the skin with extreme force

To minimise the discomfort felt by the patient always ensure that you are aware of the specific manufacturer's instructions in relation to how the drug should be injected (angle of needle and site of administration). Not following this advice will mean that you are not abiding by the licence issued for the injection, so you are giving the injection incorrectly and may be exposing the patient to unnecessary risk.

Whilst continuing to keep the skin pinched up, press the syringe plunger down to inject the medication smoothly and slowly, at a rate of 1 ml over 10 seconds. Once all of the medication has been injected quickly remove the needle and then release the pinched up skin
To ensure the medication is administered into the subcutaneous tissue.

To minimise the discomfort felt by the patient.

As soon as you have removed the needle from the patient, activate the needle safety device, if present, which will automatically cover the needle. Dispose of the needle and syringe in the sharps bin and any other equipment as per local policy. If necessary cover the injection site with a spot plaster
To reduce the chance of accidental needle stick injury.

To maintain nurse and patient safety.

Some injection sites may leak a very small amount of fluid or blood.

Remove gloves and perform hand hygiene
To reduce the chance of infection.

If PPE is required because the patient is in isolation put on a new pair of gloves.

After the medication administration has been completed ensure the patient is in a comfortable position with drinks and call bells available as necessary
Promotes patient comfort and ensures they are well nourished and hydrated.

Discard PPE, any single use equipment and other used materials as per policy. Clean any equipment used as per the relevant policy every time it is used and perform hand hygiene
To prevent cross infection and maintain equipment in working condition.

Recording administration and outcome

1 **Record that the medicine has been administered on the Medication Administration Record to ensure a legal record of the medicine administered**

You must make a clear, accurate and immediate record of all medicine administered, or any intentionally withheld or refused by the patient. You must ensure your signature is clear and legible. Ensure the registered nurse supervising you countersigns your signature.

Evaluation of the impact and effectiveness of the medication and assessment of any untoward events

1 **Monitor the effectiveness of the medication and any reactions, reporting these to a registered nurse and the medication prescriber and instigating treatment as appropriate**

Ensure you are fully aware of the therapeutic uses of the medicine to be administered, its normal dosage, side effects, precautions and contraindications. Adverse reactions to medications can range from giving discomfort to being life threatening. By administering a medicine you undertake to ensure that you are aware of any possible reactions and you know what to do in response.

Ensure you advise patients' of any signs to watch out for and identify how they can inform you.

 2 **Document relevant information on the patient's observation chart and/or in the patient's notes as necessary**
Maintains patient safety and accurate records.

Source: Adapted from Hall (2018)

Administering an intramuscular injection

☑ Essential equipment

Drug to be administered, sterile swab (to open ampoule), blunt fill needle (to draw up drug, with a filter if drawing up from a glass ampoule), safety needle (to give drug – often 21G, but choice depends upon patient and drug to be given), appropriately sized syringe, alcohol swab (for skin preparation according to local policy), injection tray (or similar), gloves, sharps bin, gauze (or similar) to apply pressure to injection site, spot plaster (or similar) to cover injection site.

Medicine Administration Record.

☑ Field specific considerations

Refer to Administering medication (pp. 67-75).

It is not uncommon for both adults and children to be very worried about having an injection. Make sure you take time to relax the patient as much as is possible and answer any questions they have. The patient may wish to have another person they trust present for the procedure (or it might be necessary to have the assistance of another member of the healthcare team or a play specialist) to hold their hand and distract their attention by, for example, talking, story-telling, singing etc.

With children local anaesthetic cream is often applied prior to the procedure. The intramuscular injection route is often used when nursing children, with the exception of immunisations and in emergency situations.

☑ Care setting considerations

It is possible for an intramuscular injection to be administered in all care settings.

☑ What to watch out for and action to take

Refer to Administering medication (pp. 67-75).

Intramuscular injections are given into the skeletal muscle. As blood flow to muscle is good, any medication given by this route will be absorbed more rapidly than if it is given orally or by a subcutaneous injection, but not as quickly as an intravenous injection.

When administering an injection ensure that you always adhere to all of the relevant policies outlined by the healthcare provider and your educational institution.

There are four sites that can be used for an intramuscular injection. The site chosen will depend upon the volume of medication to be given and how thick it is, plus the amount of muscle tissue the patient has at the injection site. The site to be used should be decided upon after consideration of these factors and take into account the patient's preference.

Deltoid

A site that is easy to access, but the muscle is small and only suitable for the administration of 1-2 mls of drug (depending upon how well developed the muscle is). There is also risk of injury to the axillary nerve in particular, plus other nerves and blood vessels in the area.

Dorsogluteal

This is the most frequently used site in adults, where up to 3 mls of drug can be administered.

The dorsogluteal site is contraindicated in children. There is the possibility of causing damage to the sciatic nerve when using this site, which can cause pain or paralysis that may be permanent. The position of the superior gluteal artery also makes inadvertent arterial drug administration a potential risk, as is accidental subcutaneous drug administration if the wrong needle choice is made in patients with larger amounts of subcutaneous tissue. Tissue necrosis, gangrene, pain, muscle contraction and fibrosis have all been associated with intramuscular injections in this site in children.

Vastus lateralis

An easy to access site, with few major blood vessels in the area. The site can be used to administer up to 2 mls of drug. Using this site can, however, cause pain and the depth of subcutaneous tissue will vary between patients.

Ventogluteal

This site provides the greatest thickness of gluteal muscle which can take up to 3 mls of drug. As there are no nerves or blood vessels in this area and the layer of subcutaneous tissue is thin, it is the preferable site for an intramuscular injection. Despite these positive factors, however, it is not frequently used in practice in the UK.

The evidence supporting the need to decontaminate the skin prior to administering an intramuscular injection is debated, so ensure that you follow the policy of the healthcare provider. If alcohol swabs are used, ensure you leave the site to dry, as alcohol can inactivate medication.

☑ **Helpful hints**

- Gloves and aprons must be worn if contact with blood/body fluids/ excreta is anticipated or the patient is in isolation.
- Gloves must be worn for all invasive procedures and all activities carrying a risk of exposure to blood, body fluids, or to sharp or contaminated instruments.
- Gloves should be worn if contact with the medication is potentially harmful to the nurse.
- Hand hygiene must be performed before touching a patient, before clean/aseptic procedures, after body fluid exposure/risk, after touching a patient and after touching a patient's surroundings.
- Waste should be disposed of in a clinical waste bag if it is contaminated with blood/body fluids/excreta.

Intramuscular injection guidelines

Ensuring safe and effective storage and administration of medication to patients

 Remember that as a nursing student you need to be supervised at all times by a registered nurse when administering medication
To ensure patient safety and support your learning.

 Identify an appropriate place to check the patient's medication, away from interruptions and distractions
To ensure patient safety as interruption is associated with medication error.

 Before you give any medication you will need to complete an assessment of your patient's medication needs. This involves:

   a   Checking the patient's care plan for specific requirements
   b   Checking the Medicine Administration Record to determine the correct medicine to be given by intramuscular injection to the correct patient, taking account of all eight rights of medicine administration.

To ensure patient safety.
    You need to be aware of the patient's plan of care to ensure no changes have been made and that the medication administration remains appropriate.

To ensure the drug is administered accurately and safely.

Medicines must be given in a timely manner in order to ensure optimum benefits from treatments.

It is dangerous to administer a medication which does not have a specific licence for a particular route.

Decide if there is any reason not to administer the intravenous injection at this time and record and report accordingly
If there has been a change in the patient's condition a medication may no longer be appropriate.

Ensure the drug to be administered by intramuscular injection is:

a   In date
b   The correct dose for the prescription
c   The correct medicine according to the prescription.

The quality of an out of date medicine may have deteriorated.

To prevent error and ensure the best possible outcome in terms of patient care.

To ensure safe practice as medicines are available in different strengths.

You must check that the prescription is clearly written and the medication is the same to ensure patient safety.

You must never give a medicine without being certain that the dosage (relating to the patient's weight where appropriate), the method of administration, the route and the timing are all correct.

If your patient is a child or the drug dose has been calculated taking account of the patient's weight, check that the prescribed dose is correct for the patient's current weight or BMI
Children's medicines are calculated on the basis of milligrams per kilogram per day.

Some adult drugs are prescribed at a dose which takes account of the patient's weight.

To ensure patient safety the dose must be checked, using an accurate patient weight.

Some specialised children's areas use BMI and surface area for drug doses. A calculator for this can be found at the BNF for children online at https://bnf.nice.org.uk

Gather the equipment required, including the needles and a syringe of the appropriate size for the amount of medication to be injected. Ensure that all packaging is intact and not past its expiry date

To ensure safe administration of the drug and safe disposal of the sharps once the medication has been administered.

 Wash your hands with soap and water. Apron and gloves should only be worn if appropriate
It may be necessary to wear gloves and an apron during the preparation of some medications.

Wearing apron and gloves as part of personal protective equipment (PPE) is a standard infection control procedure when dealing with body fluids or patients in isolation.

Ensure your use of PPE such as gloves and disposable aprons is appropriate by considering the individual patient situation and the risk presented.

 Injections should be prepared in a clean area using an aseptic non-touch technique. Attach a blunt fill needle to the syringe. Make sure you use one with a filter if you are drawing a drug up from a glass ampoule
To reduce the risk of infection.

To reduce the risk of glass particles being drawn up with the medication.

 If the drug is in a glass ampoule, flick it to remove any medication from the top. Cover the top of the ampoule with a sterile swab and snap it off along the score lines at the neck. Check that there are no particles of glass in the medication; if there are, use a new ampoule
To ensure all medication is drawn up from the ampoule.

To remove the medication safely from the ampoule.

To ensure the medication given to the patient does not contain glass.

 Draw the medication up into the syringe. Holding the syringe upright, with the needle at the top, tap the side of the syringe. Expel the air and any excess medication, leaving the correct dose in the syringe
To encourage any air bubbles to rise so they can be expelled.

 Remove the fill needle and dispose of it in the sharps bin. Attach the safety needle to be used to administer the medication using a non-touch technique
To ensure safety.

A 21G safety needle (normally green) is frequently chosen to administer medication intramuscularly. The choice however will depend upon the size of the patient and how viscous the medication is.

13 **Place the syringe on the injection tray with the other equipment and take it to the patient with the Medicines Administration Record. Ensure a sharps bin is to hand**
To enable safe administration of the medication and safe disposal of sharps.

14 **Introduce yourself to the patient, explain the procedure and gain their consent. Ensure that you adapt your communication style to meet the needs of the individual patient and their family or carers as relevant**
Every effort should be made to explain the procedure in terms that the patient can understand. This is not only respectful of their individual human rights, but also helps to ensure that they will be more accepting of the treatment and that their anxieties are reduced.

All patients should be offered the opportunity to be involved in decisions relating to their medicines at the level they wish.

For patients who are unable to provide consent because they are unconscious advice should be sought.

15 **Clear sufficient space within the environment where the drug will be administered. Place the injection tray containing the syringe in a safe place where you can see it at all times**
Enables clear access for the patient and the nurse to safely administer the medication.

To ensure patient safety whilst you complete the next step.

16 **Complete the final checks, which always include patient identity and allergies but may also include specific checks for individual drugs. Provide the patient with necessary information regarding their medication, using appropriate means of communication to aid explanation**
To ensure patient safety you must:

a   Be certain of the identity of the patient to whom the medicine is to be administered

b   Check that the patient is not allergic to the medicine before administering it

c   Before administering some drugs, cardiac ones for example, it is necessary to check that the patient's heart rate or blood pressure is not too low.

Patients, their families and carers need to be aware of the main features of the medicines given and how to manage them effectively and concordantly. They need to know what to do if the medicine is taken inappropriately and the implications of not taking it.

Decide which injection site is to be used. Ensure the patient is fully prepared for the administration of the intramuscular injection and is in an appropriate position (see next step). An infant may need to be held securely. Ask and/or assist the patient to remove their clothing as is necessary to expose the injection site (see step 19)
Offer the patient the opportunity to be involved in this decision as is appropriate.
   Patients should be in a position which ensures both comfort and safety.
   Ensure you maintain the patient's dignity and privacy.

Ensure patient is in a comfortable position that enables access to the chosen site.

Deltoid site

Seat the patient, although they may wish to stand.

Dorsogluteal site

Position the patient lying on their side to expose the chosen buttock.

Vastus lateralis site

Position the patient lying on their back.
May also be given in the sitting position, which may reflect patient preference.

Ventrogluteal site

Position the patient either lying on their back or side, or they may wish to stand.

19 **Locate the exact injection site to ensure injection is given into muscle identified**

Deltoid site

To make it easier to locate the deltoid muscle expose the patient's arm and shoulder, asking them to place their arm across their abdomen.

Dorsogluteal site

To make it easier to locate the dorsogluteal muscle ask the patient to bend up their knees.

Vastus lateralis site

To make it easier to locate the vastus lateralis muscle expose the patient's leg.

Ventrogluteal site

To make it easier to locate the ventrogluteal muscle ask the patient to bend up their knee on the chosen side.

20 **Perform hand hygiene and put on gloves**
To reduce the chance of infection.
    Gloves must be worn for all invasive procedures and all activities carrying a risk of exposure to blood, body fluids or to sharp or contaminated instruments.

21 **Remove the cover from the needle of the syringe, taking care not to contaminate it**
To ensure the needle is not contaminated.

22 **Hold the syringe like a pencil in the hand you write with. Ensure the needle is pointing towards the patient. Use the thumb of your other hand to stretch the skin over the injection site by 2 to 3 cm**
This technique is known as Z-tracking, which reduces pain and leaking from the injection site.
    You may see variations in the practice of registered nurses – some will use Z-tracking and others may not. It is always important

to ensure that you follow the drug manufacturer's recommendations and are aware of the relevant research evidence. In this way you can be certain that you give the injection correctly.

 Whilst continuing to stretch the skin, quickly insert the needle all the way into the skin at an angle of 90 degrees. Do not push the needle into the skin slowly or stab the needle into the skin with extreme force

To minimise the discomfort felt by the patient.

To ensure the muscle is reached and the medication is not administered into the subcutaneous tissue.

 Whilst continuing to stretch the skin, if you are using the dorsogluteal site check for any 'flashback', by pulling back on the plunger of the syringe. If blood enters the syringe, withdraw the needle and start the procedure again. There is no need to undertake this step with the deltoid, vastus lateralis or ventrogluteal site

Flashback describes blood entering the syringe. It is not necessary to do this with the deltoid or vastus lateralis sites, as there are few major blood vessels in these areas.

If blood is drawn back into the syringe the needle is in a blood vessel and if you administered the medication it would enter the blood supply.

These other sites do not have the risk of the needle entering a blood vessel.

 Whilst continuing to stretch the skin, slowly press the syringe plunger down to inject the medication smoothly and slowly at a rate of 1 ml per 10 seconds

To minimise the discomfort felt by the patient.

Administering the medication slowly will allow the muscle fibres to stretch in order to make space for the fluid being injected.

 Whilst continuing to stretch the skin, once all of the medication has been injected, wait 10 seconds before quickly removing the needle. When the needle has been removed, release the stretch being applied to the skin

This allows the medication to disperse evenly.

Releasing the stretch is the final part of the Z-tracking process, which prevents the fluid from leaking out of the injection site.

As soon as you have removed the needle from the patient, activate the needle safety device, if present, which will automatically cover the needle. Dispose of the needle and syringe in the sharps bin and any other equipment as per local policy. If necessary apply pressure to the injection site with dry gauze and cover with a spot plaster
To maintain nurse and patient safety.

Some injection sites may leak a very small amount of fluid or blood.

To reduce the chance of accidental needle stick injury.

Remove gloves and perform hand hygiene
To reduce the chance of infection.

If PPE is required because the patient is in isolation put on a new pair of gloves.

After the medication administration has been completed ensure the patient is in a comfortable position with drinks and call bells available as necessary
Promotes patient comfort and ensures they are well nourished and hydrated.

Discard PPE, any single use equipment and other used materials as per policy. Clean any equipment used as per the relevant policy every time it is used and perform hand hygiene
To prevent cross infection and maintain equipment in working condition.

Recording administration and outcome

Record that the medicine has been administered on the Medication Administration Record to ensure a legal record of the medicine administered
You must make a clear, accurate and immediate record of all medicine administered, or any intentionally withheld or refused by the patient. You must ensure your signature is clear and legible. Ensure the registered nurse supervising you countersigns your signature.

Evaluation of the impact and effectiveness of the medication and assessment of any untoward events

Monitor the effectiveness of the medication and any reactions, reporting these to a registered nurse and the medication prescriber and instigating treatment as appropriate

Ensure you are fully aware of the therapeutic uses of the medicine to be administered, its normal dosage, side effects, precautions and contraindications.

Adverse reactions to medications can range from giving discomfort to being life threatening. By administering a medicine you undertake to ensure that you are aware of any possible reactions and you know what to do in response.

Ensure you advise patients of any signs to watch out for and identify how they can inform you.

Document relevant information on the patient's observation chart and/or in the patient's notes as necessary

Maintains patient safety and accurate records.

Source: Baillie (2014); BNF (2021); Lister et al. (2020); National Prescribing Centre (n.d.); NICE (2017); NMC (2018); RCN (2013); Shepherd (2018); Westbrook et al. (2010); WHO (2009, 2014). Adapted from Hall (2018)

ASSISTING PEOPLE WITH THEIR NUTRITIONAL NEEDS

KATE GOODHAND AND JANE EWEN

Common steps for all nutrition-related skills

☑ Essential equipment

Depends on skill but is likely to include one or more of the following: utensils, crockery with or without adaptations, plate guard, slip mat, napkin/disposable clothes protection.

☑ Field-specific considerations

When caring for a person with a learning disability, it is important to know their level of understanding so that consent for and cooperation with the care can be gained. You will need to allow time to explain what you are doing and whether it will cause discomfort or pain.

People who have mental health problems may not understand why you need to undertake nutrition-related tasks. They may also be so depressed that they don't have the energy to eat, or those with cognitive impairment may have forgotten to eat. They may withhold consent to have their measurements taken and you may need to refer to the Mental Capacity Act 2005/Adults with Incapacity Act (Scotland 2000) and maintain their best interests.

Children have a different anatomy and physiology to adults, which varies from birth through to adolescence. You will need knowledge of paediatric anatomy and physiology to enable you to interpret the results. As younger children may not understand why you need to undertake the task, you will need to modify your approach. It is usually helpful to have parents or carers present to assist.

☑ **Care-setting considerations**

In hospital or a care home, seek the person's preference for eating alone or in company. At home, individuals may need food and drink prepared and served by healthcare workers.

☑ **What to watch out for and action to take**

While undertaking any nutrition-related skill, you should also assess:

- the person's position
- their neurological condition – are they alert and responsive?
- any signs or complaints of pain or discomfort
- the views of the person or their relatives' views – these may provide you with important additional information.

The information gained from these observations will enable you to fully assess their condition, institute appropriate treatment as necessary and escalate care needs to senior nurses and the medical team.

☑ **Helpful hints**

- The correct personal protective equipment (PPE) should be worn.
- Hand hygiene must be performed before touching a patient, after touching a patient and after touching a patient's surroundings.
- Waste should be disposed of in a clinical waste bag.

Nutrition guidelines

The first step of any procedure is to introduce yourself, explain the procedure and gain the person's consent
Fully informed consent may not always be possible if you are caring for a child or if the person has mental health problems or learning disabilities, but even in these circumstances, every effort should be made to explain the procedure in terms that they can understand.

This is not only respectful of their individual human rights, but also helps to ensure that they will be more accepting of the treatment and that their anxieties are reduced.

For people who are unable to provide consent because they are unconscious, advice should be sought from your practice educator or another qualified nurse.

 Gather the equipment required (see individual skills for equipment required). Ensure these are clean and in working order
Reduces the chance of infection and maintains patient and nurse safety.

 Clear sufficient space within the environment, for example around the bed space or chair
Enables clear access for the patient and the nurse to safely use the equipment required.

 Wash your hands with soap and water before you start the task. Don the correct PPE
Ensure your use of PPE is appropriate by considering the individual's situation and the risk presented.

 Ask them if they wish to have the curtains drawn for privacy or to be in a separate room
Some people may feel exposed.
Maintain their privacy, dignity and comfort as required.

 The person needs to be in a comfortable position, either sitting in a chair, resting on a couch or in bed and well supported
Promotes comfort and reduces anxiety.

 After performing the task, ensure they are in a comfortable position, with drinks and call bells available as necessary
Promotes comfort and ensures they are well nourished and hydrated and ensures patient safety.

 Discard PPE, any single-use equipment and other used materials as per policy. Clean any equipment used as per the relevant policy every time it is used and perform hand hygiene
Prevents cross-infection and maintains equipment in working condition.

 Document findings on their food and fluid observation chart and/or in the patient's notes
Maintains patient safety and accurate records.

10 **If any changes are observed, escalate to senior nursing staff/ your practice educator immediately**

It is vital to report any changes to a registered nurse immediately so they can ensure care is escalated.

Source: Lister et al. (2020); WHO (2009)

Weighing a patient

☑ What is normal

Most adults will know their height but often get their weight wrong!
Refer to the BMI chart to determine if weight is in proportion to height.

☑ Before you start

Remember the common steps (Nutrition guidelines, pp. 96–98).

☑ Essential equipment

Appropriate weighing scales:

- 0–2 years – baby scales
- over 2 years – sitting or standing scales
- for patients with mobility needs – hoist scales.

☑ Field-specific considerations

When caring for someone with a learning disability, it is important to know their level of understanding so that consent for and cooperation with the measurement can be gained. You will need to allow time to explain what you are doing and why.

People who have mental health problems may not understand why you need to undertake nutrition-related skills, or may simply require further details, full explanation and reassurance.

If you are weighing a child, prepare them by using an age-appropriate explanation (you may use a play specialist to assist). If possible, involve the child's parents or carers to reassure the child. If a child becomes upset, do not weigh them, but document the reason and return later.

☑ **Care-setting considerations**

People can be weighed in any care setting, if the scales are in working order and accurately calibrated.

☑ **What to watch out for and action to take**

While undertaking any nutrition-related task, you should also assess:

- the patient's positioning and ability to mobilise
- their neurological condition - are they alert and responsive?
- any signs or complaints of pain or discomfort
- the patient's or relatives' views, as these may provide you with important additional information.

The information gained from these observations will enable you to fully assess the person's condition, institute appropriate treatment as necessary and escalate needs care to senior nurses and the medical team.

Weighing guidelines

1 **Perform steps 1-6 of the Nutrition guidelines (pp. 96-97)**
To prepare the person and yourself to undertake the task.

2 **Remove clothing as appropriate:**

- 0-2 - remove clothing.
- Over 2 - remove shoes or slippers, and empty pockets; light indoor clothing should be worn.

To reduce the chance of abnormal readings.

3 **Ensure scales are calibrated, on a flat surface, can be accessed easily and the dial is on zero, and apply brakes if appropriate**
If the scales are the 'stand on' type, ensure the patient stands on the scales centrally, with feet slightly apart, and keeps still without holding onto anything.
    To ensure patient safety and promote accuracy of the reading.

Perform steps 7-10 of the Nutrition guidelines (pp. 97-98)
To ensure that:

- the patient is safe, comfortable, and receiving the appropriate care
- the results have been documented in the patient's records
- the equipment is clean and in working order.

Source: Best and Shepherd (2020); Lister et al. (2020); RCN (2017)

Assisting a patient to eat and drink

☑ What is normal

It is normal for patients, children included, to eat and drink with only minimal assistance, so remember to enable the patient to be as independent as possible.

☑ Before you start

Remember the common steps (Nutrition guidelines, pp. 96-98).
Check the patient's plan of care to ascertain whether there is a known swallowing difficulty.

☑ Essential equipment

- clean table or tray (and a chair for you to sit on)
- utensils - adapted if appropriate
- crockery and any necessary adapted items, such as a plate guard
- clothing protection for the patient, such as disposable covers or napkins, as required
- the meal and a suitable drink
- field-specific considerations

When caring for a patient with a learning disability, ascertaining their likes and dislikes is imperative to maintaining nutritional needs.
Many mental health conditions can affect appetite and the ability to prepare food as well as to eat and drink normally, so extra support may be required.

For children, age-appropriate food and choice of utensils are important safety issues.

Elderly patients may not eat or drink adequately due to problems with dentures and oral hygiene, plus the accessibility of food, or because of the effects of medication.

☑ Care-setting considerations

It is possible to assist a patient to eat and drink in any care setting. In community settings, you may need to involve other agencies to help a patient maintain adequate nutrition throughout the whole day.

☑ What to watch out for and action to take

If the patient seems to have any difficulty swallowing at any time, stop immediately and report your concerns straight away to your practice educator or another registered nurse.

When assisting a patient to eat or drink, you should also assess:

- the patient's positioning and ability to mobilise
- their neurological condition – are they alert and responsive?
- any signs or complaints of pain or discomfort
- the patient's or relatives' views, as these may provide you with important additional information.

The information gained from these observations will enable you to fully assess the patient's condition, institute appropriate treatment as necessary and escalate needs care to senior nurses and the medical team.

Eating and drinking assistance guidelines

Perform steps 1-6 of the Nutrition guidelines (pp. 96-97)
To prepare the patient and yourself to undertake the skill.

Prepare the patient for the meal by:

- offering toilet and hand-washing facilities before the meal arrives
- ascertaining where the patient wishes to eat and that the patient is in as upright a position as possible

- if using a bed table, removing surplus equipment, particularly items such as sputum pots and vomit bowls
- cleaning the table and ensuring it is at the correct height
- collecting the correct diet for the patient and the utensils they require
- ensuring you have a supply of fresh water or appropriate fluid.

To empower the patient and reduce infection risks.

A social environment is often preferred to encourage normality, but some may wish to eat alone.

To promote an environment conducive to eating and drinking.

To ensure everything is to hand so you do not have to leave the patient.

Position yourself close to the patient, at the same level as them, in a comfortable position
To promote the patient's dignity and ensure you are in a position that protects your back.

Ensure the patient approves of the food choice and that food is at an appropriate temperature and consistency
To empower the patient and prevent harm from heat or swallowing difficulties.

Offer as much or as little assistance as is required. While assisting the patient, ensure pace is correct by asking for feedback. Ensure you offer food in the order the patient wishes, following their preferences. Wait until they have swallowed the food before offering any more
Communicate appropriately with the patient while they are eating, to make the experience a sociable and enjoyable one; avoid asking the patient questions when they have a mouthful of food.

To empower the patient while promoting autonomy and dignity.

Remember to offer and encourage fluids at frequent intervals while the patient is eating. Take care when offering hot drinks that they are at a suitable temperature
To aid swallowing and promote digestion; avoid burning the patient.

Ensure the patient is not rushed and has sufficient time to complete their meal. Encourage the patient to eat but do not pressurise them if they indicate they have had enough to eat
To ensure the patient eats and drinks the amount they wish.

8 Clear away crockery and utensils; offer patient appropriate hygiene, such as handwashing, mouth care, clean dentures and clean bed table
To promote patient comfort and a clean environment.

9 Leave patient in a comfortable, upright position for at least 30 minutes, with their call bell to hand
To promote digestion and ensure patient safety.
For children, this will depend on their condition and stage of development, but in general aim to disturb the child as little as possible after feeding and encourage quiet activities for a while.

10 Perform steps 7–10 of the Nutrition guidelines (pp. 97–98)

Source: Lister et al. (2020); NICE (2012b); RCN (2011)

Passing a nasogastric tube

☑ What is normal?

Many patients who we care for will be able to maintain their own nutrition and fluids, however some patients may need additional help. When this is necessary it is essential we follow the NICE (2012b) quality standards for nutritional support in adults. There are two ways we can provide nutrition for patients who can't swallow safely. A nasogastric tube can be passed or a gastrostomy created. There are advantages and disadvantages to both methods. A nasogastric tube is inserted quickly and easily, however they need replacing frequently and patient acceptance is often poor (NICE, 2012b). If the tube is going to be used for feeding it is crucial the position of the tube is ascertained correctly to avoid inadvertent placement in the lungs, which if undetected can have fatal consequences.

☑ Before you start

Remember the common steps for all care delivered to assist patients.

☑ Essential equipment

- clinically clean tray/receptacle
- fine bore nasogastric tube – adult 6 FG–10 FG / introducer

- syringe 50 ml (catheter tip or luer slip to fit end of tube)
- disposable cup 3/4 full with tap water – to lubricate nasogastric tube
- cotton buds/tissue
- universal pH indicator paper/strips
- disposable gloves – non-sterile
- hypoallergenic adhesive tape
- denture bowl – where required
- disposable paper sheet
- glass of iced water if not contraindicated.

☑ Field specific considerations

If assisting a patient who has a learning disability/any cognitive impairment or a child, it is important to ascertain their level of understanding. In these cases it may be appropriate to have parent(s) or carers present to help reassure the patient.

☑ Care setting considerations

Can be in any care setting: acute, rehabilitation, community hospital or home. NICE (2012b) sets out quality standards. These include standards for carers who manage nasogastric tubes.

☑ What to watch out for and action to take

Correct preparation and positioning of the patient can help you pass the nasogastric tube safely. If an obstruction is felt when introducing into the nose try the other nostril. Seek help from a colleague if in doubt. If a patient shows signs of distress (gasping or cyanosis) stop the procedure immediately and remove the tube. Always check the position of the tube before use as displaced tubes can be fatal.

☑ Helpful hints

- Gloves and aprons must be worn as contact with body fluid is anticipated.
- Hand hygiene must be performed before touching a patient, before clean/aseptic procedures, after body fluid exposure/risk, after touching a patient and after touching a patient's surroundings.
- Waste should be disposed of in a clinical waste bag if it is contaminated with blood/body fluids/excreta.

Passing a nasogastric tube guidelines

 Perform steps 1-6 of the Nutrition guidelines (pp. 96-97)
To prepare the patient and yourself to undertake the skill.

 As you explain the procedure also arrange a signal by which a patient can tell you that they need you to stop (e.g. raising hand)
So patient feels they have some control - this should help to reduce anxiety.

 Request/assist the patient to sit in a semi-upright position in the bed or chair. Support the patient's head with a pillow. The unconscious or dense hemiplegic patient should be placed flat in bed with one pillow under the head
To allow for an easier passage of the tube.
This position enables swallowing and ensures that the epiglottis is not obstructing the oesophagus.

 Clean the patient's nostrils, if required. Encourage the patient to sniff with one nostril closed at a time
This is to make the procedure more comfortable for the patient and removes any obstructions/ensures patency of the nasal cavity.

 Request the patient to/remove their dentures (if appropriate) and place in denture bowl
This is so you do not displace dentures with the tube.

 Protect the patient's clothing with a disposable paper sheet
To maintain patient dignity and comfort.
To minimise the risk of cross infection.

 Wash and dry hands again
To prevent cross infection.

 Put on gloves
To protect hands from body fluids.

Holding the nasogastric tube, estimate the distance from the patient's ear lobe to the bridge of the nose and then to the lower end of the xiphisternum, without making contact with the skin or patient's clothing

Research (Taylor et al., 2014) indicates that the NEX (nose-ear-xiphisternum) measurement may not be long enough to reach the stomach, so this is only a guide. They suggest adding 10 cm but state ONLY an EM trace or direct vision would be conclusive.

To provide an indication of the length of tube required to reach the patient's stomach.

 Follow manufacturer's instructions regarding visual checks and recommendations if using a guide wire

To ensure safe effective use of the equipment.

 Dip the tube in water (do not use lubricating gel as it gives an acid reaction)

To activate the external lubricant thus reducing friction between the mucous membrane and the tube.

 Gently insert the tube through the nostril and slowly advance it along the nasal passage. If an obstruction is felt, withdraw slightly then advance the tube again at a slightly different angle. Gentle rotation of the tube can be helpful

To facilitate passage of the tube by following the natural anatomy of the nose.

 Request the patient to swallow as the tube is advanced. Sips of iced water may be offered to facilitate this unless contraindicated

To facilitate closure of the epiglottis enabling the tube to pass into the oesophagus.

 Continue to advance the tube until the length required has been passed. If an obstruction is felt do not force, withdraw the tube slightly and attempt to reinsert, or withdraw completely and repass, or try another nostril

To maintain patient safety.

Secure the tube to the cheek using hypoallergenic adhesive tape and hook over the ear

To maintain the tube in position and keep it out of the patient's visual field and avoid friction to the nose/prevent allergic reaction. Change tape daily and use alternate sides of nose to prevent from becoming sore.

Confirm tube is in the stomach by withdrawing gastric content and checking on pH indicator paper/strips and/or perform a chest/upper abdominal x-ray
Please refer to your local policy for guidance.

To ensure the tube is correctly placed in the stomach – wrongly placed or falsely verified tubes can be fatal.

Fill a syringe with 10 ml of tap water and slowly flush the tube. Gently remove the guide wire from the tube and discard
NOTE: Once the position has been confirmed remove the guide wire. To remove the guide wire attach an enteral dispenser (syringe) containing 10 mls of water to the end of the tube and slowly inject the water down the tube. This activates the internal lubricant in the tube and aids removal.

The tube should be held firmly at the tip of the nose to ensure that the tube stays in position as the guide wire is removed. The guide wire should never be reinserted while the tube is still in the patient.

To facilitate the easy removal of the guide wire from the tube. Remember to always check the position of the tube before flushing as aspiration pneumonia can be caused if the tube is misplaced in the lungs and pH testing may be affected leading to a false positive reading (NPSA, 2012).

Measure all the visible tube from the tip of the nose and record in patient documentation
To provide a record to help detect if the tube has moved (NPSA, 2011). Accurate record keeping promotes patient safety (NMC, 2018).

Clean dentures if removed. Either replace or leave in bowl with clean water
For patient oral hygiene and comfort.

Perform steps 7-10 of the Nutrition guidelines (pp. 97-98)
To ensure that:

- the patient is safe, comfortable and receiving the appropriate care
- results have been documented in the patient's records
- any equipment is clean and ready to be reused.

Source: NICE (2012b); NPSA (2011, 2012); NMC (2018)

Confirmation of position of a nasogastric tube

☑ What is normal?

The position of a fine bore nasogastric tube should always be checked:

- after initial placement
- before commencing feed
- prior to administration of medicines if feed not in progress
- at least once daily if on continuous feeds
- after vomiting, excessive coughing, prolonged hiccoughing or oro-pharyngeal suction
- when there is any suggestion of tube displacement
- if there are any new or unexplained respiratory sounds.

☑ What to watch out for and action to take

Following an evidence-based review in 2011 by NPSA only two methods can confirm the gastric position of a nasogastric tube - the pH of the tube aspirate and an x-ray, and that x-ray should only be a second line if no aspirate and pH reading is obtained. Check your local policy for guidance.

If a nasogastric tube is not tolerated, perhaps due to poor patient compliance, then discuss with multidisciplinary team and consider creation of a gastrostomy.

☑ Essential equipment

- clean tray
- syringe (50 ml)
- universal pH indicator paper/strips (only pH strips with a clear CE mark should be used (NPSA, 2011))
- disposable gloves - non-sterile
- nasogastric tube position confirmation record or nasogastric tube placement checklist if tube has been placed/replaced.

Confirmation of position of nasogastric tube guidelines

(1) **Perform steps 1-6 of the Nutrition guidelines (pp. 96-97)**
To prepare the patient and yourself to undertake the skill.
To minimise the risk of cross infection.

2 **Attach new clean 50 ml syringe to nasogastric tube and withdraw plunger to obtain gastric content. Detach syringe from nasogastric tube**

If no aspirate obtained use these techniques recommended in the NPSA (2011) decision tree:

Adults

- If possible turn an adult onto left side.
- Inject 10–20 ml air through the tube and then gently withdraw plunger. Wait 15–30 minutes before aspirating again.
- Advance or withdraw tube by 20 cm.

Children/infants (not neonates) (NPSA, 2011)

- Inject 1–5 ml into the tube using a syringe.
- Wait for 15–30 minutes before aspirating again.
- Advance or withdraw tube by 1–2 cm.

All

- Give mouth care to nil orally patients.
- Do not use water to flush until tube position confirmed.

It is recognised that obtaining aspirate from fine bore tubes can be difficult.

This stimulates gastric secretion of acid.

 3 **Put small amount of aspirate onto pH indicator paper/strip**
To prevent harm to patient.

 4 **Compare indicator paper to colour and check pH acceptable to commence use of tube**
A pH of 1 to 5.5 indicates that the tube is positioned correctly and is safe to use. However if the reading has a pH of 5 to 6, then a second competent person should check the result and/or retest.

5 **If unable to confirm position by aspirate then an x-ray will be necessary**
A pH of 6 or above could indicate misplacement of the tube and should not be used (NPSA, 2011). To avoid false readings tubes MUST NOT be flushed with water prior to confirming position (NPSA, 2012).

6 **The method of confirming position should always be documented with the pH obtained where appropriate**
Accurate record keeping promotes patient safety (NMC, 2018).

7 **Perform steps 7-10 of the Nutrition guidelines (pp. 97-98)**
To ensure that:

- the patient is safe, comfortable and receiving the appropriate care
- results have been documented in the patients records
- any equipment is clean and ready to be reused.

Source: NMC (2018); NPSA (2011, 2012)

Maintaining a nasogastric tube

☑ What is normal?

Nasogastric tubes are prone to displacement and care is required to ensure they are retained in the correct positon. Skin condition should be monitored carefully as the tube and tape can cause sores.

☑ Before you start

Remember the common steps for all care delivered to assist patients.

☑ Essential equipment

- patient's toiletries
- bowl of water
- towel
- shaver (if required)
- tissues
- hypoallergenic tape
- mouthwash
- vomit bowl (to rinse out mouth).

☑ Field specific considerations

If assisting a patient who has a learning disability/any cognitive impairment or a child, it is important to ascertain their level of understanding. In these cases it may be appropriate to have parent(s) or carers present to help reassure the patient.

☑ Care setting considerations

Can be in any care setting: acute, rehabilitation, community hospital or home.

☑ What to watch out for and action to take

Red sore areas around ears and nose. Change tape and positon of tube regularly.

☑ Helpful hints

- Gloves and aprons must be worn as contact with body fluid is anticipated.
- Hand hygiene must be performed before touching a patient, before clean/aseptic procedures, after body fluid exposure/risk, after touching a patient and after touching a patient's surroundings.
- Waste should be disposed of in a clinical waste bag if it is contaminated with blood/body fluids/excreta.

Maintaining a nasogastric tube guidelines

Nasal hygiene:

Gently clean area. Encourage patient to blow nose if necessary.

Change position of tube exit site ensuring tape not pulling tube too tightly.

To allow nostrils to remain unblocked.

To prevent pressure sore.

Oral hygiene:

Regular oral hygiene with mouthwashes.

Encourage patient to brush teeth and gums regularly.

Patient often breathes with nasogastric tube in situ so the mouth can become dry.

If patient on nil by mouth then saliva may not be produced as normal.

Facial cleansing:

Daily removal of tape and normal face washing.

Avoid use of moisturiser where tape is to be applied.

Area around tube often neglected for fear of disturbing tube.

Excess oils can make it difficult to secure tape.

Shaving as normal for men

Promote patient-centred care.

Changing tape:

Carefully remove all old tape before applying new.

Skin condition below tape should be checked.

Tape can lose its adherence qualities.

Prevent damage to skin.

Flushing for maintenance:

Tube should be flushed before and after use.

To ensure that tube remains patent.

Source: Lister et al. (2020)

Removing a nasogastric tube

☑ What is normal?

It is normal to replace nasogastric tubes every 10-28 days depending on the type of tube and material it is made from; always follow the manufacturer's guidelines (NICE, 2012b).

☑ Before you start

Remember the common steps for all care delivered to assist patients.

☑ Essential equipment

- clean tray
- tissues
- disposable gloves - non-sterile
- disposable paper sheet
- polythene bag.

☑ Field specific considerations

If assisting a patient who has a learning disability/any cognitive impairment or a child, it is important to ascertain their level of understanding. In these cases it may be appropriate to have parent(s) or carers present to help reassure the patient.

☑ Care setting considerations

Can be in any care setting: acute, rehabilitation, community hospital or home.

☑ Helpful hints

- Gloves and aprons must be worn if contact with blood/body fluids/ excreta is anticipated or the patient is in isolation.

- Hand hygiene must be performed before touching a patient, before clean/aseptic procedures, after body fluid exposure/risk, after touching a patient and after touching a patient's surroundings.
- Waste should be disposed of in a clinical waste bag if it is contaminated with blood/body fluids/excreta.

Removing a nasogastric tube guidelines

Perform steps 1-6 of the Nutrition guidelines (pp. 96-97). Wash hands and put on gloves
To prepare the patient and yourself to undertake the skill.
   To minimise the risk of cross infection.

Protect patient's clothing with a disposable paper sheet
To promote patient dignity and protect clothing.

Remove tape securing tube. If nasal bridle is in situ please cut tape above clip
To allow tube to move freely.

Pinch tube and gently withdraw tube into polythene bag
To prevent spillage on removal through oesophagus.

Give patient tissue to clean nasal area/blow nose
Promote patient comfort and dignity.

Perform steps 7-10 of the Nutrition guidelines (pp. 97-98)
To ensure that:

- the patient is safe, comfortable and receiving the appropriate care
- the results have been documented in the patient's records
- any equipment is clean and ready to be reused

Source: NICE (2012b); NMC (2015)

Caring for a PEG (pertcutaneous endoscopic gastronomy)*

*This skill relates to patients who have a well established PEG tube site.

☑ What is normal?

Healthy individuals consume food and fluids by eating and drinking. Food and fluids are taken orally and begin the process of digestion in the mouth. Some patients are required to receive fluid and nutrition via a PEG tube, an example being someone who has had a stroke and can no longer swallow. PEG tube sites should be cleaned daily. Some patients may be self-caring and will do this whilst showering or bathing.

☑ Before you start

Remember the common steps for all care delivered to assist patients.

☑ Essential equipment

- suitable personal protective equipment: in this case, gloves and apron are sufficient
- bactericidal alcohol hand gel
- soap and warm water
- gauze swabs and/or cotton buds
- towel (or something to dry the skin)
- dressings (if applicable).

☑ Field specific considerations

If assisting a patient who has a learning disability, it is important to ascertain their level of understanding.

As is appropriate depending upon the age of a child, encourage and assist parents or carers to become involved in care to maintain as far as is possible their normal caring role.

☑ Care setting considerations

PEG tube care may occur in any care setting.

☑ What to watch out for and action to take

This procedure could be considered to be intimate and may cause the patient embarrassment or distress. Ensure you promote the patient's dignity and provide privacy at all times.

☑ Helpful hints

- Gloves and aprons must be worn if contact with blood/body fluids/excreta is anticipated or the patient is in isolation.
- Hand hygiene must be performed before touching a patient, before clean/aseptic procedures, after body fluid exposure/risk, after touching a patient and after touching a patient's surroundings.
- Waste should be disposed of in a clinical waste bag if it is contaminated with blood/body fluids/excreta.

PEG guidelines

Perform steps 1-6 of the Nutrition guidelines (pp. 96-97). Position the patient for the procedure
To prepare the patient and yourself to undertake the skill.
To allow ease of access, maintain patient comfort and to adhere to moving and handling regulations.

Remove any dressings which may be in situ
To allow inspection of the PEG tube site.

Examine the skin around the PEG tube looking for:

- redness/inflammation/swelling/foul smelling odour
- discharge
- encrustation
- excess skin tissue development.

To assess for signs of infection, leakage from the site or granulation tissue (a recognised minor complication). If any of these are present, seek advice from your practice educator or other registered nurse/healthcare professional.

Clean the site with warm soap and water, using swabs/cotton buds to gently remove any encrustation which may have developed
To cleanse the skin.

Rinse the area
To remove any soap/residue which may cause skin irritation.
Powders or creams should be avoided as this may cause skin irritation.

Dry the area thoroughly, using cotton buds to dry under the PEG tube
To prevent any deterioration of the skin.

Apply any prescribed creams/ointments
For therapeutic effect.

Apply dressing if required
To protect the PEG tube site.
Dressings should only be needed if there is continued discharge.

Perform steps 7-10 of the Nutrition guidelines (pp. 97-98)
To ensure that the:

- patient is safe, comfortable and receiving the appropriate care
- results have been documented in the patient's records
- any equipment is clean and ready to be reused.

Source: Simons and Remington (2013)

Stoma care

☑ **Essential equipment**

Suitable appliance (stoma pouch or bag), scissors, measuring guide, gloves and apron, access to sink or bowl of warm water, wipes, measuring jug if required, receptacle for soiled disposable items.
Appliances come as a one piece closed system, one piece drainable system or a two piece system.

☑ **Care setting considerations**

Always ensure you have the equipment required to safely meet the patient's needs in your current setting. For example, in a community setting it may be necessary to dispose of waste in the rubbish bin. This should be double bagged first.

The size of the appliance is determined by measuring the stoma using the measuring device that accompanies the appliances. Some appliances need to be cut to size. Too large an opening in the bag exposes the skin to the bag contents and too small an opening may cause trauma to the stoma.

☑ What to watch out for and action to take

Whilst maintaining stoma care be aware of:

- the colour of the stoma and surrounding skin
- the consistency of the faeces
- any complaints of pain or discomfort.

The information gained from these observations will enable you to fully assess the condition of the patient's skin and if necessary plan any changes in treatment plus evaluate whether the current treatment is effective. Any abnormalities or changes must be reported to a relevant individual and recorded in the patient's notes.

☑ Field specific considerations

It is important to ascertain what a patient's usual routine is, as children or patients with a learning disability or cognitive impairment may not be able to tell you. Assisting a patient to develop their ability to maintain their elimination needs can be an important step towards independence.

Patients who are severely depressed may not view stoma care as important, so both physical and psychological support could be required.

Encourage and assist parents or carers to be involved to maintain the usual routine. Supporting, educating and enabling parents or carers to adopt new care practices within any environment is an important nursing role.

Stoma care guidelines

1 **The first step of any procedure is to introduce yourself to the patient, explain the procedure and gain their consent**
There will be differences in how you go about this for children or those with mental health or learning disabilities as not all patients will be able to provide consent, but they will be able to assent.

It could be that the procedure is one normally undertaken by the patient's family or carer, or they may express the wish to be involved in the care you are about to deliver. If this is so, and it is appropriate, it is an opportunity to maintain the patient's usual routine, or you could support the patient's family or carer in adapting their usual routine to meet the patient's changed care needs.

 Gather the equipment required. Ensure these are clean as appropriate
To ensure you are ready to complete the procedure.

 Ensure privacy, so close doors and curtains/blinds as necessary. If you are at a patient's bed space ensure you draw the curtains fully
Patients will need to feel comfortable when carrying out stoma care.
Maintains privacy, dignity and comfort.
Caring for a patient's hygiene is a personal and intimate procedure which takes time to perform with dignity.

 Ensure the patient is in a comfortable position; adjust clothing to expose the abdomen
To ensure the area is visible for the patient to access or to observe.

 Wash your hands, put on an apron and gloves
To prevent contamination from body fluids.

 As appropriate encourage the patient to undertake as much of the process as possible
Promotes independence.

 Place disposable wipes around stoma site
To protect surrounding skin from spills or leakage.

 Empty the appliance and if necessary measure contents
To monitor output and to ensure easier removal.

 Remove appliance and dispose of in a disposable bag or receptacle
To ensure safe disposal.

Wash skin surrounding the stoma with warm water and wipes
To remove excess faeces and ensure skin is intact.

11 Observe surrounding skin for signs of redness and excoriation and also colour and condition of stoma
To ensure complications are identified promptly.

 12 Dry skin thoroughly around stoma site and apply barrier wipes or sprays
To prevent excoriation and to ensure the new appliance will be securely attached.

 13 Prepare appliance and place in position
Ensure appliance is prepared as per manufacturer's guidelines. This will ensure skin is protected.

 14 Dispose of any waste products as per guidelines
To ensure safe disposal.

 15 Remove your apron and perform hand hygiene and document in the patient's notes the care you have given and any relevant observations of pressure areas etc.
Reduces the risk of infection.

 16 Offer support for the patient and ensure the patient is comfortable
Maintains patient safety and accurate records.

Source: Baillie (2014); Lister et al. (2020); NMC (2018)

Peripheral vascular cannula care

☑ **What is normal?**

Many patients who are cared for in an in-patient environment such as an acute hospital will have an intravenous peripheral cannula inserted. This device is usually located in the back of the hand or forearm but occasionally may be sited in other places such as the foot. It is used to provide intravenous medications and/or fluids. Blood samples may be obtained at the time of insertion but that should not be the only reason for inserting a cannula. Cannulas should be removed if no longer required.

☑ Before you start

Remember the common steps for all care delivered to assist patients. This procedure uses the aseptic non-touch technique; make sure you are familiar with it.

☑ Essential equipment

- suitable personal protective equipment, in this case, gloves and apron are sufficient
- bactericidal alcohol hand gel
- a clean trolley or surface for your equipment
- sterile dressing pack (containing sterile swabs) and normal saline
- antiseptic solution (as per local policy)
- transparent dressing (as per local policy)
- sharps bin (may be required).

☑ Field specific considerations

If assisting a patient who has a learning disability, it is important to ascertain their level of understanding.

As is appropriate depending upon the age of a child, encourage and assist parents or carers to become involved in care to maintain as far as is possible their normal caring role.

Reassurance may be required as some patients may associate peripheral vascular cannula care with the pain/discomfort of having the cannula inserted in the first place.

☑ Care setting considerations

Predominantly in an in-patient care setting.

☑ What to watch out for and action to take

Infection is a risk when patients have a peripheral vascular cannula in situ; be aware of what the common signs and symptoms of infection are and report anything abnormal to your practice educator or other registered healthcare professional.

☑ Helpful hints

- Gloves and aprons must be worn if contact with blood/body fluids/ excreta is anticipated or the patient is in isolation.

- Hand hygiene must be performed before touching a patient, before clean/aseptic procedures, after body fluid exposure/risk, after touching a patient and after touching a patient's surroundings.
- Waste should be disposed of in a clinical waste bag if it is contaminated with blood/body fluids/excreta.

Peripheral vascular cannula care guidelines

Perform steps 1-6 of the Nutrition guidelines (pp. 96-97)
To prepare the patient and yourself to undertake the skill.

Position the patient for the procedure
To allow ease of access, maintain patient comfort and to adhere to moving and handling regulations.

Remove any dressings which may be in situ
To allow inspection of the cannula site.

Examine the skin around the cannula looking for: redness/ inflammation/swelling/discharge/bleeding
To assess for signs of infection.
    If any of these are present, seek advice from your practice educator or other registered nurse/healthcare professional.

Clean the site with sterile swabs and normal saline, being careful not to dislodge the cannula
To cleanse the skin and remove any residue which may cause skin irritation.

Dry the area thoroughly
To prevent any deterioration of the skin.

Scrub the port(s) of the cannula using an antiseptic solution containing 70% isopropyl alcohol for 15 seconds or more (or as per local policy)
To remove any microbial contamination and reduce the risk of infection.

Apply sterile, transparent dressing (as per local policy)
To allow visual inspection of the cannula site and reduce the risk of mechanical phlebitis. Do not secure with a bandage as this prevents the site from being observed.

Perform steps 7-10 of the Nutrition guidelines (pp. 97-98)
To ensure that:

- the patient is safe, comfortable and receiving the appropriate care
- results have been documented in the patient's records
- any equipment is clean and ready to be reused.

Source: Health Protection Scotland (2014); Lister et al. (2020); McCallum and Higgins (2012); NMC (2018)

ASSISTING PEOPLE WITH THEIR ELIMINATION NEEDS

MAIREAD COLLIE, DAVID J. HUNTER AND VALERIE FOLEY

Common steps for all elimination-related skills

☑ **Essential equipment**

Depends on skill but is likely to include one or more of the following:

- suitable personal protective equipment (PPE)
- bedpan and paper cover, urinal, commode
- toilet paper
- equipment to enable the patient to wash their hands
- manual handling equipment and possibly assistance from another member of the healthcare team
- soap and warm water, single-use washcloths and towels.

☑ **Field-specific considerations**

When caring for a patient with a learning disability, it is important to know their level of understanding so that consent for and cooperation with the care can be gained. You will need to allow time to explain why you are doing the measurements and whether they will cause discomfort or pain.

Patients who have mental health problems may not understand the relevance of the care you plan to deliver. They may therefore withhold consent and you may need to refer to the Mental Capacity Act 2005, or the Adults with Incapacity (Scotland) Act 2000, and best interest.

When assisting children with elimination needs, if possible it is usually helpful to have the parents or carers present to assist.

☑ Care-setting considerations

Assisting patients with elimination needs can occur within all settings, although you may not have all the equipment available to assist you. For example, in a patient's home you may not have manual handling equipment, so to ensure patient safety and your own, thorough risk assessments need to be undertaken.

☑ What to watch out for and action to take

While assisting a patient with their elimination needs, as appropriate, you should also observe and assess:

- the condition of their skin
- their ability to move or mobilise independently
- their neurological condition – are they alert and responsive?
- any signs or complaints of pain or discomfort
- the patient's or relatives' views – for example, saying that their needs have changed or that they are experiencing problems
- any changes reported by the patient regarding the colour, smell and consistency of their urine and any changes in their stool.

The information gained from these observations will enable you to fully assess the patient's condition and institute appropriate treatment as necessary.

☑ Helpful hints

- Gloves and aprons must be worn if contact with blood/body fluids/ excreta is anticipated or the patient is in isolation.
- Hand hygiene must be performed before touching a patient, before clean/aseptic procedures, after body fluid exposure/risk, after touching a patient and after touching a patient's surroundings.
- Waste should be disposed of in a clinical waste bag if it is contaminated with blood/body fluids/excreta.

The first step of any procedure is to introduce yourself to the patient, explain the procedure and gain their consent
Fully informed consent may not always be possible if the patient is a child or has mental health problems or learning disabilities, but even in these circumstances, every effort should be made to explain the procedure in terms that the patient can understand. This is not only respectful of their individual human rights, but also helps to ensure that they will be more accepting of the treatment and that their anxieties are reduced.

For patients who are unable to provide consent because they are unconscious, advice should be sought from your practice educator or another qualified nurse.

Gather the equipment required (see individual skills for equipment required). Ensure these are clean as appropriate and in working order
Ensures the skill is performed effectively.

Reduces the chance of infection and maintains patient and nurse safety.

Clear sufficient space within the environment, for example around the bed space or chair
Enables clear access for the patient and the nurse to safely use the equipment required.

Wash your hands with soap and water before you start any care activity. Apron and gloves should only be worn if appropriate
Wearing an apron and gloves as part of PPE is a standard infection-control procedure when dealing with body fluids or patients in isolation.

Ensure your use of PPE such as gloves and disposable aprons is appropriate by considering the individual patient's situation and the risk presented.

Ensure you promote patient dignity and privacy as appropriate, for example by drawing curtains or moving the patient to a bathroom if at all possible
Elimination needs are intimate and personal. At all times you need to maintain patient privacy, dignity and comfort as required.

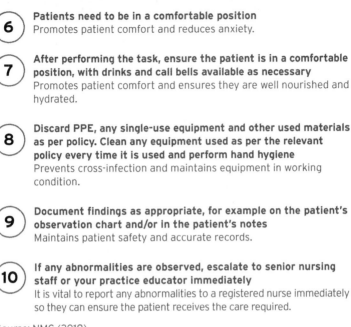

6 Patients need to be in a comfortable position
Promotes patient comfort and reduces anxiety.

7 After performing the task, ensure the patient is in a comfortable position, with drinks and call bells available as necessary
Promotes patient comfort and ensures they are well nourished and hydrated.

8 Discard PPE, any single-use equipment and other used materials as per policy. Clean any equipment used as per the relevant policy every time it is used and perform hand hygiene
Prevents cross-infection and maintains equipment in working condition.

9 Document findings as appropriate, for example on the patient's observation chart and/or in the patient's notes
Maintains patient safety and accurate records.

10 If any abnormalities are observed, escalate to senior nursing staff or your practice educator immediately
It is vital to report any abnormalities to a registered nurse immediately so they can ensure the patient receives the care required.

Source: NMC (2018)

Assessing bowel function

☑ What is normal?

'Normal' bowel function can vary greatly: some patients open their bowels daily, others every 2 or 3 days. If possible, it is best to ask the patient what is 'normal' for them and whether they take laxatives.

☑ Before you start

Remember the common steps for all care delivered to assist patients with their elimination needs (Elimination assistance guidelines, pp. 126-127).

Remember to review any documentation regarding the patient and update any relevant care plans. Other factors need to be considered when assessing a patient's bowel function, as this will enable you to assess the patient's overall condition. As you approach the patient, observe them carefully to assess whether they are well nourished and hydrated. Do they look in good health or do they appear unwell, and are they able to move unaided?

☑ **Essential equipment**

Relevant documentation with regard to bowel assessment. This can vary between patients depending on the field, as well as between care settings. Appropriate PPE.

☑ **Field-specific considerations**

If assessing a patient who has a learning disability, it is important to ascertain their level of understanding. If appropriate, involve a family member or carer in the discussion.

When assessing a patient with mental health problems, their level of capacity may need to be considered, so they may require support and assistance to enable them to recognise that they are constipated.

As appropriate depending on the age of a child, encourage and assist their parents or carers to become involved, as they will provide useful information.

☑ **Care-setting considerations**

An assessment of bowel function can be undertaken in any care setting.

☑ **What to watch out for and action to take**

Remember that the questions you are going to ask may cause anxiety and embarrassment.

If any abnormalities are found, this must be reported to a qualified nurse immediately and recorded in the patient's notes.

Bowel function assessment guidelines

1 **Perform steps 1-6 of the Elimination assistance guidelines (pp. 126-127)**
To prepare the patient and yourself to undertake the task.

Document the history of the present bowel complaint
To gain an understanding of the patient's needs and to direct management or treatment decisions.

Undertake a holistic assessment of the patient's condition, which includes details of their diet, fluids, mobility, dexterity, cognitive function and usual environment
To obtain a comprehensive and holistic assessment which may identify the underlying reason for the patient's altered bowel habit, whether constipation or diarrhoea.

Document the patient's usual bowel pattern
To ascertain what is 'normal' for the patient.

Ask the patient what medications they are currently taking
To assess if medication has affected the normal bowel routine.

Ask the patient to identify their stool formation using the Bristol Stool Chart
To enable clear identification of the patient's needs and allow for effective management.

As is appropriate within the care setting, ensure that future bowel actions are monitored and accurately recorded
To monitor condition and detect abnormalities.

Develop a plan of care in partnership with the patient and their parents or carers as appropriate
To produce a clear plan of care to be delivered to the patient and ensure that the patient is aware of and happy with the ongoing management of the condition.

Perform steps 7-10 of the Elimination assistance guidelines (p. 127)
To ensure that:

- the patient is safe, comfortable and receiving the appropriate care
- the results have been documented in the patient's records.

Source: NMC (2018)

Assisting a patient to use a bedpan, urinal or commode

☑ What is normal?

Female patients may need to use a bedpan or commode to both micturate and defecate; male patients may prefer to micturate in a urinal, which may be easier if they stand up (if this is appropriate).

☑ Before you start

Remember the common steps for all care delivered to assist patients with their elimination needs (Elimination assistance guidelines, pp. 126-127).

☑ Essential equipment

- appropriate PPE
- appropriate bedpan and paper cover or commode or urinal and paper cover
- toilet paper
- facilities to allow the patient to wash their hands
- manual handling equipment as required
- possible assistance from a further member of the healthcare team.

☑ Field-specific considerations

If assisting a patient who has a learning disability or cognitive impairment, it is important to ascertain their level of understanding.

As appropriate depending on the age of a child, encourage and assist parents or carers to become involved in care to maintain their normal caring role as far as is possible.

☑ Care-setting considerations

A patient can be assisted to use a bedpan, commode or urinal in any care setting.

☑ What to watch out for and action to take

Elimination is an intimate and personal activity. Ensure you promote the patient's dignity and provide privacy at all times.

(1) **Perform steps 1-6 of the Elimination assistance guidelines (pp. 126-127)**
To prepare the patient and yourself to undertake the task.

(2) **Bedpan or urinal**
Assess the moving and handling needs of the patient.

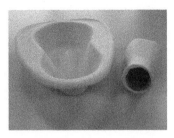

(3) **Comode**
Assess the moving and handling needs of the patient. Ensure the patient's weight does not exceed the manufacturer's recommendations.

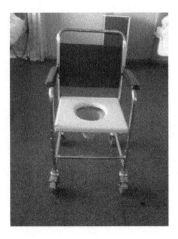

To maintain a safe environment and to determine whether or not additional assistance is required.

Remove the bedclothes and, if the patient is able, assist them to sit upright. Ask the patient (or use moving and handling equipment if required) to raise their hips/buttocks to allow the bedpan or urinal to be correctly positioned. If the patient cannot raise their hips/buttocks, a rolling motion may be used with appropriate moving and handling techniques to roll the patient onto the bedpan

Support with pillow if required.

Take the equipment to the bedside, checking that the wheels on the commode are secured and that there is a bedpan receiver placed under the commode.

Remove the commode cover and assist the patient to transfer from bed/chair to the commode. Ensure the patient is comfortable.

A comfortable position may make it easier for the patient to open their bowels.

To ensure patient safety.

When the patient is on the bedpan or has the urinal in position, ask them to move their legs slightly apart so that you can check the position is correct

Check the patient is positioned correctly on the commode.

Checking the position will reduce the risk of spillage and associated contamination or cross-infection.

If safe to do so, leave the patient, ensuring that toilet paper is close at hand and giving them a nurse call button. Cover the patient's legs with a towel or sheet

This step is not possible if you are supporting a patient to use a urinal while standing.

To maintain privacy and dignity.

When the patient has finished using the bedpan, commode or urinal, you may need to assist them with personal hygiene. As indicated, select the appropriate PPE and clean the patient's bottom using toilet paper, wiping from front to back. Skin cleanser or warm soapy water may be required

Assisting the patient to be clean will ensure patient comfort.

Wiping from front to back will reduce the spread of infection from the bowel to the urethra (especially in female patients).

Pat the skin dry after assisting the patient with their personal hygiene
To prevent deterioration of the patient's skin.

Help the patient to wash and dry their hands
To promote patient comfort, dignity and infection control.

Perform steps 7-10 of the Elimination assistance guidelines (p. 127)
To ensure that:

- the patient is safe, comfortable and receiving the appropriate care
- the results have been documented in the patient's records
- any equipment is clean and ready to be reused.

Source: Ballentyne and Ness (2009); NMC (2018); Oxford University Hospitals NHS Trust (2016)

Performing catheter care

☑ What is normal?

Catheter care should be undertaken as a part of the patient's routine hygiene care.

☑ Before you start

Remember the common steps for all care delivered to assist patients with their elimination needs (Elimination assistance guidelines, pp. 126-127).

☑ Essential equipment

- appropriate PPE
- soap and warm water
- single-use washcloths
- towel.

☑ **Field-specific considerations**

If assisting a patient who has a learning disability, it is important to ascertain their level of understanding.

As appropriate depending on the age of a child, encourage and assist parents or carers to become involved in care to maintain their normal caring role as far as is possible.

☑ **Care-setting considerations**

Catheter care can be undertaken in any care setting.

☑ **What to watch out for and action to take**

Performing catheter care is an intimate and personal activity. Ensure you promote the patient's dignity and provide privacy at all times.

Catheter care guidelines

Perform steps 1–6 of the Elimination assistance guidelines (pp. 126-127)
To prepare the patient and yourself to undertake the task.

Assist the patient to be correctly positioned for the procedure
To allow ease of access, maintain patient comfort and adhere to moving and handling regulations.

Clean the genital area using soap and water
Soap and water are appropriate; anti-bacterial or antiseptic solutions are not required.

Perform meatal cleansing:

a   In male patients by pulling back the foreskin (if uncircumcised). Note that the foreskin should not be forcibly pulled back. It can take until the late teenage years before the foreskin can be retracted

Clean around the glans, moving away from the meatal opening; clean the area where the catheter enters the penis and then downwards along the catheter.

Rinse and dry the area.

Return the foreskin to the original position.

b　In female patients by gently parting the labia

Clean the area where the catheter enters the meatus and then downwards along the catheter.

Rinse and dry the area.

To reduce the risk of spreading infection.

To expose the glans penis and the urethral meatus.

To reduce contamination.

To remove any buildup of smegma.

To reduce the risk of irritation from soap and to maintain skin integrity.

To reduce the risk of paraphimosis developing.

To expose the inner genitals (labia minora) and the urethral meatus.

To reduce contamination, particularly from the anus.

To reduce the risk of irritation from soap and to maintain skin integrity.

Make sure that the area is completely dry
To reduce the risk of skin breakdown. Talcum powder should be avoided as irritation may be caused.

Ensure that the patient is comfortable and re-dressed following the procedure
To promote patient comfort and dignity.

Perform steps 7-10 of the Elimination assistance guidelines (p. 127)
To ensure that:

- the patient is safe, comfortable and receiving the appropriate care
- the results have been documented in the patient's records
- any equipment is clean and ready to be reused.

Source: Hunter (2012); Leaver (2007); NMC (2018)

Emptying a patient's catheter bag

☑ What is normal?

Catheter bags should only be emptied when they are full, as each time you perform this procedure you are potentially introducing an infection risk.

☑ Before you start

Remember the common steps for all care delivered to assist patients with their elimination needs (Elimination assistance guidelines, pp. 126-127).

Do not forget that a catheter bag is attached to a patient and that you need to ask for their consent to perform this procedure.

☑ Essential equipment

- appropriate PPE
- alcohol swabs
- sterile jug or disposable container.

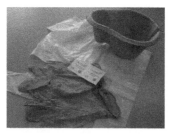

☑ Field-specific considerations

If assisting a patient who has a learning disability, it is important to ascertain their level of understanding.

As appropriate depending on the age of a child, encourage and assist parents or carers to become involved in care to maintain their normal caring role as far as is possible.

☑ Care-setting considerations

Emptying a catheter bag can be undertaken in any care setting.

☑ What to watch out for and action to take

Emptying a catheter bag can be seen by patients to be the same activity as using the toilet. Ensure you promote the patient's dignity and provide privacy at all times. If the patient's urine output is not being monitored frequently and you notice when emptying the bag that the patient has passed little or no urine, check the patient's fluid balance chart, as their catheter bag may have just been emptied. If this is not the case, you must inform your practice educator or a registered nurse, as it may indicate a problem relating to catheter drainage or an alteration in the patient's condition. Patients who are catheterised may have an overnight drainage bag attached, which will be removed when the patient mobilises and be replaced with a leg bag.

Catheter care guidelines

 Perform steps 1–6 of the Elimination assistance guidelines (pp. 126–127)
To prepare the patient and yourself to undertake the task.

 Clean the outlet port of the catheter bag with the alcohol swab and allow to fully dry
To reduce the risk of infection.

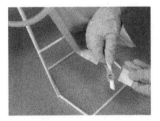

 Open the port and allow the urine to drain into the jug

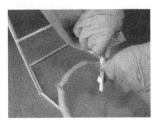

To empty the bag and, if required, to allow measurement of the volume of urine passed.

Close the port and clean again with an alcohol swab

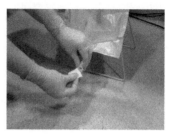

To reduce the risk of infection.

Reposition the catheter bag and check that the patient is comfortable
To ensure the patient is comfortable.

Cover the jug and transfer to the sluice where the urine can be disposed of. If required, the urine should be measured
To reduce the risk of contamination.
    To monitor the patient's condition and to maintain accurate documentation.

Perform steps 7–10 of the Elimination assistance guidelines (p. 127)
To ensure that:

- the patient is safe, comfortable and receiving the appropriate care
- the results have been documented in the patient's records
- any equipment is clean and ready to be reused.

Source: NHS Greater Glasgow and Clyde (2017); NMC (2018)

Urinalysis

☑ **Before you start**

Remember the common steps for all care delivered to assist patients with their elimination needs (Elimination assistance guidelines, pp. 126–127).
  Assess the colour and smell of the urine.

☑ **Essential equipment**

White-top sterile specimen containers or bedpans are the most commonly used receptacles. To undertake accurate urinalysis, the receptacle needs to be clean but not necessarily sterile, so any clean receptacle which can hold water may be used.

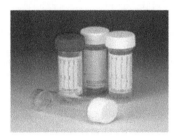

☑ **Care-setting considerations**

Can be measured in any care setting.
  Ensure that the patient has the mobility necessary to use the commode, urinal or bedpan. If this is not the case, offer assistance and support and apply safe patient moving techniques. Catheterisation may be considered, but the need for this would be carefully risk-assessed.

Specimen collection guidelines

 Perform steps 1–5 of the Elimination assistance guidelines (p. 126)
To prepare the patient and yourself to undertake the task.

Ensure the container you are going to use to obtain the specimen is appropriately labelled with the patient's identification details
To ensure that you test the correct specimen.

First voided morning urine is best suited for urinalysis
Its concentration provides the most reliable results.

It is best to test specimens immediately; if not possible, then do so within 2 hours
This provides the most reliable results.

After shaking the sample, briefly completely immerse the whole section of the strip where the test pads are located into freshly voided urine
Shake the sample to ensure it is mixed so the concentration will be constant throughout.

Dip the strip briefly to avoid dissolving out reagents from the test pads which would produce incorrect results.

As you remove the strip from the sample, run its edge against the edge of the receptacle – apply the 'dip and drag' stages of the 'dip, drag, blot, read' technique (see figure below)
To remove excess urine and prevent the strip from dripping.

Hold the strip horizontally
To avoid potential mixing of reagents due to them running down the strip. This would cause cross-reactions that will produce unreliable results.

Remove excess urine by applying the 'blot' stage of the 'dip, drag, blot, read' technique (see figure below)
Blot the edge of the strip on absorbent material such as a paper towel. Take care not to touch the test pads and maintain the strip in a horizontal position.

To prevent the strip from dripping.

Compare all test pads with the corresponding colour chart. At the time specified, record all results
This is the 'read' stage of the 'dip, drag, blot, read' technique (see figure below). Make sure that when you are comparing the test pads with the corresponding colour, you do not hold the strip

directly against the container, as there may be urine remaining on the strip which you would transfer to the container.

It is important to follow the timings specified to ensure that your results are correct. Colour changes that have occurred after 2 minutes are invalid and will not provide accurate results.

Perform steps 8-10 of the Elimination assistance guidelines (p. 127)
To ensure that:

- the patient is safe, comfortable and receiving the appropriate care
- the results have been documented in the patient's records.

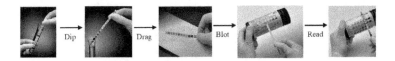

Source: Smith and Roberts (2011)

ASSISTING PATIENTS WITH THEIR HYGIENE NEEDS

CATHERINE DELVES-YATES

Common steps for all hygiene procedures

☑ **Essential equipment**

Depends on skill but is likely to include one or more of the following:
Single-use bowls, warm water, towels, soap, incontinence pads, disposable washcloths, skin moisturiser or talc (if the person wishes), clean clothes, nightwear or gown, clean bedlinen.

☑ **Field-specific considerations**

When assisting an individual with a learning disability, it may be important to ascertain what their usual hygiene routine is, as they may not be able to tell you. Assisting a person to develop their ability to maintain their hygiene needs can be an important step towards independence.

Individuals with mental health problems – who are severely depressed, for example – may not view their personal hygiene as important, so both physical and psychological support could be required. People with a cognitive impairment such as dementia or psychosis may not realise or even understand what is needed.

When caring for a child, encourage and assist parents or carers to be involved in hygiene care to maintain the usual routine. Supporting, educating and enabling parents or carers to continue their care within any environment is an important nursing role.

☑ Care-setting considerations

It is not always possible to have all the equipment available to assist an individual to safely meet their hygiene needs in the exact manner they wish. For example, in a person's home you may not have a hoist, so it may not be safe for them to use their bath; however, you can still assist them to meet their hygiene needs in a different way.

Always ensure you have the equipment required to safely meet the person's needs in your current setting.

☑ What to watch out for and action to take

While maintaining an individual's hygiene, you should assess:

- the colour of the skin, lips, nail beds and sclera of their eyes
- the location and appearance of any rashes
- whether the skin is dry and/or flaky
- the condition of pressure areas, for any bruises, open areas, pale or reddened areas; the appearance of any wounds and whether or not they are draining
- any complaints of pain or discomfort
- the temperature of the person's skin.

The information gained from these observations will enable you to fully assess the condition of the individual's skin and, if necessary, plan any changes in treatment, plus evaluate whether the current treatment is effective.

☑ Helpful hints

- Gloves and aprons must be worn if contact with blood/body fluids/excreta is anticipated or the person is in isolation.
- Hand hygiene must be performed before touching any individual, before clean/aseptic procedures, after body fluid exposure/risk, after touching a person and after touching a person's surroundings.
- Waste should be disposed of in a clinical waste bag if it is contaminated with blood/body fluids/excreta.
- Equipment must be cleaned as identified by the relevant policy every time it is used.

The first step of any procedure is to introduce yourself to the person, explain the procedure and gain their consent
Fully informed consent may not always be possible if the individual is a child or has mental health problems or learning disabilities, but even in these circumstances, every effort should be made to explain the procedure in terms they can understand. This is not only respectful to them as a person, but also helps to ensure they will be more accepting of the treatment and that their anxieties are reduced.

For individuals who are unable to provide consent because they are unconscious, advice should be sought from your practice supervisor or another qualified nurse.

It could be that the procedure is one normally undertaken by the individual's family or carer, or they may express the wish to be involved in the care you are about to deliver. If this is so, and if it is appropriate, it is an opportunity to maintain the person's usual routine, or you could support their family or carer in adapting their usual routine to meet any changed care needs.

 Gather the equipment required (see relevant skill for details)
Ensure these are clean as appropriate.

Reduces the chance of infection and maintains the safety of all involved.

 Clear sufficient space within the environment, for example in the bathroom or around the bed space
Enables clear access for all involved to safely use the equipment required.

Wash your hands and put on an apron. Gloves should only be worn if absolutely necessary, never 'just in case'
Wearing gloves creates a barrier between the nurse and the individual being cared for as it sends signals that the nurse is undertaking 'dirty tasks'.

Wearing an apron and gloves as part of personal protective equipment (PPE) is a standard infection-control procedure when dealing with body fluids or people in isolation.

Ensure your use of PPE such as gloves and disposable aprons is appropriate by considering the individual situation and the risk presented.

Ensure privacy, so close doors and curtains/blinds as necessary. If you are at a person's bed space, ensure you draw the curtains fully. Assist the individual to find a comfortable position and ensure they will not get cold

Do not hurry and be gentle.

Only expose the area of the body you need to attend to at that particular moment.

The individual being cared for will need to feel able to remove their clothing without being seen by others. Maintain privacy, dignity and comfort at all times.

Caring for an individual's hygiene is a personal and intimate procedure which takes time to perform with dignity.

Washing areas of the body can result in cooling.

Areas of the skin can be very delicate.

As appropriate, encourage the person to undertake as much of the process as possible

Promotes independence.

Equipment used for hygiene needs, such as electric shavers, must not be shared

Reduces the risk of infection.

After you have completed the hygiene procedure, remove any towels that have been used to protect the person and assist them to get into a comfortable position

Promotes comfort.

Remove your apron and perform hand hygiene. Document in the person's notes the care you have given and any relevant observations of pressure areas etc.

Reduces the risk of infection.

Maintains safety and accurate records.

10 **Offer or support the person to have a drink (so long as this is not contraindicated)**

Promotes comfort and ensures the person is well nourished and hydrated.

Source: Baillie et al. (2014); Lister et al. (2020); NICE (2017); NMC (2018); Price and McAlinden (2017); Steel (2017); WHO (2020)

Bathing a person in bed

☑ What is normal

Most people have their own hygiene practices, which may be very different from yours, so remember the stages of CLEAN to ensure you are working in partnership with those you care for.

Remember to constantly observe and assess the individual's skin. It can be more difficult to identify early changes in skin integrity in people with darkly pigmented skin, so ensure that you pay careful attention to any areas that look even slightly different in colour to those adjacent.

☑ Before you start

Remember to perform the common steps (Hygiene assistance guidelines, pp. 144–145).

☑ Essential equipment

Single-use bowl x2, warm water, towel x3, soap, incontinence pads, disposable washcloths, skin moisturiser or talc (if the individual wishes), clean clothes, nightwear or gown, clean bedlinen.

☑ Care-setting considerations

It is possible to bed-bath a person in a variety of settings as long as the necessary equipment is available.

☑ What to watch out for and action to take

If, while bed-bathing a person, you notice any areas of skin which look abnormal, this must be reported to a relevant individual and recorded in the person's notes.

Bed-bathing guidelines

1 **Perform steps 1-7 of the Hygiene assistance guidelines (pp. 144-145)**
To prepare the individual and yourself to undertake the task.

2 **Offer assistance as required to undress the person. Only uncover the area you are washing; the rest of the person should remain covered by either the bed sheets or a dry towel**
Maintains dignity and keeps the person warm.

3 **Fill a bowl with fresh warm water, check the temperature carefully and, if possible, check that the person is happy with the temperature. Change this water at any time if it becomes too cool or dirty. Always change the water after washing the perineal area and buttocks**
Aids safety.
    Reduces risk of contamination.

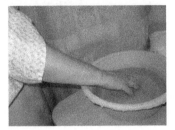

4 **Disposable washcloths are much better than a flannel for washing people as you can dispense with them when they have been used**
Always use new washcloths for the person's face, torso, back and perineal area. To keep the water as clean as possible, do not put a soapy washcloth back into the water - dispose of it and use a new one.
    Bacteria rapidly multiply in wet, warm environments such as a flannel.
    Reduces risk of contamination.

5 **Ensure the bed is at a height at which it is comfortable for you to work, changing this throughout the procedure as necessary**
Cares for your back.

6 **Start by washing the person's face. If possible, check with the individual whether they prefer to use soap for areas of their body such as their face. If you use soap, rinse it off well. Avoid getting soap in eyes**
Reduces risk of contamination.
    Prevents soap left on the skin making it dry and itchy.

7 Use a clean washcloth for each part of the body
Avoids transferring contaminants.

8 Wash each area of the person's body by wetting the washcloth
and then wringing it out to prevent dripping water. Always pat
the skin thoroughly dry with a towel. If possible, ask the person
whether they feel dry
If people are not thoroughly dried, they will become cold.

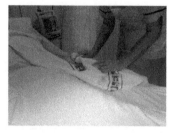

9 Once you have washed the person's face, move to the arm
furthest away from you. Place a towel underneath and wash
the hand, then arm, then armpit using soap. Take special care
to avoid any dressings or cannulae. Rinse the soap off well and
dry with the towel. Repeat the process for the other arm
Prevents dripping on areas previously washed.
   Reduces risk of infection.

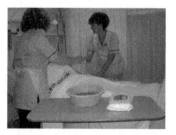

10 Next, wash the torso using soap. If the person has breasts,
gently lift them and wash underneath. Repeat this procedure
with any other skin folds that may be present. Once again, be
very careful not to get any dressings, drains or other lines wet
Rinse the soap off and dry the area thoroughly.

Skin under the breasts or skin folds needs to be cleaned and dried to avoid fungal infections.

If the person wishes, apply deodorant, moisturiser or talc. When finished, cover the torso with a dry towel
Continues the person's normal routine.
Maintains dignity and keeps the person warm.

Lift the bedsheet back to expose the person's feet and legs, but ensure you keep the genitals covered. Place a towel under the leg furthest away and wash the foot and leg with soap. Ensure you clean very gently between the toes. Rinse well. Dry thoroughly and repeat with the other foot and leg. If the person you are caring for has diabetes, ensure you assess the condition of the skin on their feet.
Prevents dripping on areas previously washed.
Maintains dignity and keeps the person warm.
Ensures that there is no evidence of diabetic foot ulcers or other skin damage in people with diabetes.

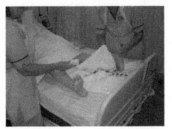

Change the water and put on gloves if you are not already wearing them
Potential contact with body fluids/excreta.

Ask the person if you can wash their genitals now and obtain their consent. Some people may wish to wash this area themselves, so offer them this opportunity
Promotes independence and maintains dignity.

The genital/perineal area is very delicate and needs special care. Wash very gently with warm water alone, rinse well and pat dry. Work from the cleanest to the dirtiest area, so from the front to back (urethral to anal area)

To wash an uncircumcised adult male, you will need to gently retract the foreskin to wash the urethral meatus. Remember to gently return the foreskin after washing to prevent swelling and discomfort. If the person is unable to do this, you will need to obtain their consent and explain exactly what you are doing while you do it.

Reduces potential of contamination.

This would not be done with a child.

If the person has a catheter, carry out the appropriate catheter care following local policy

Reduces risk of infection.

When clean and dry, re-cover the person and dispose of the water and the single-use bowl. Remove your gloves and wash your hands. Reapply gloves if necessary and refill a new single-use bowl with warm water

Maintains dignity and keeps the person warm.

Reduces risk of infection.

Even if the bedlinen is not wet or soiled, this is a good time to change it. If the person is unable to move easily in the bed, you will need another carer to assist you to change the sheets while the person is still in the bed

Ensure you abide by manual handling policies and that the bed is at the correct height, and use a slide sheet if required to reposition the person.

Promotes comfort.

Cares for your back.

Assist the person to roll onto their side, facing away from you and towards the other carer. Ensure the other carer is able to support the person and the person feels safe. Cover the person's front with the bed sheet

Ensures safety.

Maintains dignity.

Roll the old sheet into the middle of the bed and place a towel behind the person

Use soap to wash the person's back, then rinse and dry thoroughly

Keeps the person warm.

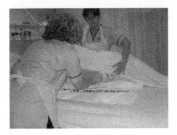

 Ask the person's consent to wash their sacral area/buttocks
If the person is soiled, put on gloves if you are not wearing them already. Wash, rinse and dry thoroughly. If appropriate, remove gloves, dispose of them and wash your hands.
Reduces risk of contamination.

 Remove towel from behind person. If sheet rolled up behind/ under person is damp or soiled, cover with an incontinence pad
Reduces risk of contamination.

 Tuck a clean sheet under mattress edge closest to you; smooth it over the mattress behind the person and roll up the part which will go under the person

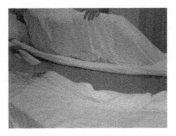

 Assist the person to roll onto their other side; remember to tell them they will roll over a bump due to the rolled sheets. Remove old sheet and incontinence pad if appropriate. Dispose of them as per policy
Reduces risk of infection.

Unroll clean sheet and tuck tightly under the mattress
Wrinkle-free sheets promote comfort.

 Assist the person to re-dress as appropriate and move into a comfortable position
Promotes comfort and dignity.

 Finish changing the bedlinen by putting clean pillowcases on the pillows, with a clean top sheet and blankets if required

(29) **Dispose of bowl or clean with detergent and water if reusable. Store inverted to avoid dregs of water collecting in it. Dispose of/ clean any other equipment as per local policy and return any of the person's equipment to their locker. Clean the bedside table and put any belongings you moved back in their original position. If appropriate, ensure the person can reach the nurse call bell**
Reduces risk of infection.
Maintains safety.

 Perform steps 8-10 of the Hygiene assistance guidelines (p. 145)
To ensure that:

- the person is safe, comfortable and receiving the appropriate care
- the results have been documented in the person's records
- the equipment is clean and in working order.

Source: Baillie et al. (2014); Black and Simende (2020); Lister et al. (2020); Price and McAlinden (2017); NICE (2017); NMC (2018); Steel (2017)

Assisting a patient with a wash (out of bed)

☑ **What is normal**

Most patients have their own hygiene practices, which may be very different from yours, so remember to ensure you are working in partnership with your patient.

Remember to constantly observe and assess the patient's skin.

☑ **Before you start**

Remember to perform the common steps (Hygiene assistance guidelines, pp. 144–145).

☑ **Essential equipment**

Single-use bowl, warm water, towels, soap, incontinence pads, disposable washcloths, skin moisturiser, talc and deodorant (if the patient wishes), clean clothes, nightwear or gown for the patient.

☑ **Care setting considerations**

It is possible to assist a patient with a wash in all settings as long as the necessary equipment is available. If it is appropriate take the patient to the bathroom. If the patient is unable to leave their bed space, clear sufficient space on their table and assist them to sit in a chair.

☑ **What to watch out for and action to take**

If whilst washing a patient any areas of skin have been observed which are abnormal this must be reported to a relevant individual and recorded in the patient's notes.

Assisting a patient with a wash guidelines

1 **Perform steps 1–7 of the Hygiene assistance guidelines (pp. 144–145)**
To prepare the patient and yourself to undertake the skill.

2 **Offer assistance as required to undress the patient. Only uncover the area you are washing; use towels to cover the rest of the patient. Assist the patient to find a comfortable position**
Maintains patient dignity and keeps them warm. If you are at the patient's bed space ensure you draw the curtains fully.

Encourage the patient to undertake as much of the process as possible to promote independence. Sitting upright makes the process of washing easier.

3 Fill a bowl with fresh warm water, check the temperature carefully and if possible check that the patient is happy with the temperature. Change this water at any time if it becomes too cool or dirty. Always change the water after washing the perineal area and buttocks

Patient safety.
    Reduces risk of contamination.

4 Disposable washcloths are much better than a flannel for washing patients as you can dispense of them when they have been used

Bacteria rapidly multiply in wet, warm environments.

5 Always use a new washcloth for the patient's face, torso, back and perineal area. To keep the water as clean as possible do not put a soapy washcloth back into the water; dispose of it and use a new one

Reduces risk of contamination.

6 Ensure the bowl and the patient are at a height at which it is comfortable for you to work, changing this throughout the procedure as necessary

Cares for your back.

7 Start by washing the patient's face. If possible check with the patient whether they prefer to use soap for areas of their body such as their face. If you use soap rinse it off well. Avoid getting soap in their eyes

Reduces risk of contamination.
    Prevents soap left on the skin making it dry and itchy.

8 Use a clean washcloth for each part of the body

Avoids transferring contaminants.

9 Wash each area of the patient's body by wetting the washcloth and then wringing it out to prevent dripping water all over the patient. Always pat the skin thoroughly dry with a towel. If possible ask the patient whether they feel dry

If patients' are not thoroughly dried, they will become cold.

10 Once you have washed the patient's face move to the arm furthest away from you. Wash the hand, then arm, then armpit using soap. Take special care to avoid any dressings or canulae. Rinse the soap off well and dry with the towel. Repeat the process for the other arm

Prevents dripping on areas previously washed.
  Reduces risk of infection.

11 Next wash the torso and back using soap. For female patients or men with gynecomastia gently lift the breasts and wash underneath. Repeat this procedure with any other skin folds that may be present. Once again be very careful not to get any dressings, drains or other lines wet. Rinse the soap off and dry the area thoroughly

Skin under the breasts or skin folds needs to be cleaned and dried to avoid fungal infections.

12 If the patient wishes, apply deodorant, moisturiser or talc. When finished cover the torso and back with a dry towel

Continues the patient's normal routine.

13 Expose the patient's feet and legs, but ensure you keep the genitals covered. Start with the leg furthest away and wash the foot and leg with soap. Ensure you clean very gently between the toes. Rinse well. Dry thoroughly and repeat with the other foot and leg

Maintains patient dignity and keeps them warm.

14 Change the water and put on gloves if you are not already wearing them

Potential of contact with body fluids/excreta.

15 Ask the patient if you can wash their genitals and sacral area and obtain their consent. Some patients may wish to wash this area themselves, so offer them this opportunity

Promotes independence and maintains dignity.

16 The genital/perineal area is very delicate and needs special care. Wash very gently with warm water alone, rinse well and pat dry. Work from the cleanest to the dirtiest area, so from the front to back (urethral to anal area). To wash an uncircumcised adult

male patient you will need to gently retract the foreskin to wash the urethral meatus. Remember to gently return the foreskin after washing to prevent swelling and discomfort. If the patient is unable to do this you will need to obtain their consent and explain exactly what you are doing whilst you do it
Reduces potential of contamination.
This would not be done with a child.

 If the patient has a catheter; carry out the appropriate catheter care in line with local policy
Reduces risk of infection

 When clean and dry re-cover the patient and dispose of the water and the single use bowl. Remove your gloves and wash your hands. Reapply gloves if necessary and refill a new single use bowl with warm water
Maintains patient dignity and keeps them warm.
Reduces risk of infection.

 Assist the patient to re-dress as appropriate and move into a comfortable position
Promotes patient comfort and dignity.

 Dispose of bowl or clean with detergent and water if reusable. Store inverted to avoid dregs of water collecting in it. Dispose of/ clean any other equipment as per local policy and return any of the patient's equipment to their locker. Clean the bedside table and put any belongings you moved back in their original position. If appropriate ensure the patient can reach the nurse call bell
Reduces risk of infection.
Maintains patient safety.

 Perform steps 8-10 of the Hygiene assistance guidelines (p. 145)
To ensure that the:

- patient is safe, comfortable and receiving the appropriate care
- results have been documented in the patient's records
- equipment is clean and in working order.

Source: Baillie (2014); Glasper et al. (2010); Lister et al. (2020); NICE (2012a); NMC (2018); Sargeant and Chamley (2013)

Shaving

☑ What is normal

Most people have their own hygiene practices, which may be very different
from yours, so remember the stages of CLEAN to ensure you are working
in partnership with those you care for.

☑ Before you start

Remember to perform the common steps (Hygiene assistance guidelines,
pp. 144-145).

☑ Essential equipment

Using an electric shaver - electric shaver, bowl, warm water, towel, mirror
and moisturiser or aftershave (if the person wishes).
   Using a safety razor - safety razor, shaving foam, bowl, warm water, dry
towel, mirror and moisturiser or aftershave (if the person wishes).

☑ Field-specific considerations

When assisting a person with a learning disability, it may be important to
ascertain what their usual shaving routine is, as they may not be able to
tell you.
   People with mental health problems - who are severely depressed, for
example - may not view their personal hygiene as important, so both
physical and psychological support could be required.

☑ Care-setting considerations

Ensure dignity is maintained as most individuals carry out all of their
hygiene practices in private.
   Shaving can be undertaken in any care setting.

☑ What to watch out for and action to take

If you observe any skin areas that are abnormal, you need to report this to
a relevant individual, record it in the person's notes and do not apply skin
moisturiser or aftershave, as this may potentially aggravate the areas. It
can be more difficult to identify early changes in skin integrity in people

with darkly pigmented skin, so ensure that you pay careful attention to any areas that look even slightly different in colour to adjacent areas.

Shaving assistance guidelines

 Perform steps 1-7 of the Hygiene assistance guidelines (pp. 144-145)
Prepares the person and yourself to undertake the task.

 Drape a towel around the person's front
Protects clothes.

 Wash the person's face and dry it thoroughly
Cleans the area, enables observation of the skin plus any shaving preferences, such as sideburns etc.

 If any of the stubble is more than 1 cm or so long, use a beard trimmer to cut this first
Long hairs will be pulled out rather than cut by an electric shaver or safety razor.

Electric shaver

a   Shave in the opposite direction to hair growth, making small circular motions if short stubble is present. For longer stubble, create larger circular motions
b   Avoid repeatedly shaving the same area

Safety razor

a   Apply shaving foam to the person's face and neck
b   Pull the area you are about to shave taut - where you start is a matter of preference
c   Angle the razor to approx. 45 degrees away from the face. Using as little pressure as possible, move the razor across the skin in the direction of hair growth
d   Repeat this process once more on the same area of skin and then move to another area
e   Frequently dip the razor into the warm water

f   If there is a large amount of stubble, you may need to use more than one safety razor

g   Rinse the person's face with cool water when you have finished shaving all areas

Results in the closest, most comfortable shave and prevents skin from becoming sore.
   Removes the hair and any excess shaving foam.

If the person desires apply moisturiser or aftershave, but remember if you use aftershave to apply it sparingly, as it can sting
Enables the continuation of usual hygiene practices.
   Do not apply moisturiser or aftershave to areas of sore or broken skin.

Assist the person to look at their face in the mirror to ensure they approve of the result
Helps the person present themselves in the manner they desire.

Perform steps 8–10 of the Hygiene assistance guidelines (p. 145)
To ensure that:

- the person is safe, comfortable and receiving the appropriate care
- the results have been documented in the person's records
- equipment is clean and in working order.

Source: Baillie et al. (2014); Black and Simende (2020); Lister et al. (2020); NICE (2017); NMC (2018)

Teeth-cleaning

☑ What is normal

Most people have their own hygiene practices, which may be very different from yours, so remember the stages of CLEAN to ensure you are working in partnership with those you care for.

☑ Before you start

Remember the common steps (Hygiene assistance guidelines, pp. 144–145).

☑ Essential equipment

Toothbrush, toothpaste, disposable cup, bowl, towel, mouthwash (if the person wishes) and mirror.

☑ Field-specific considerations

When assisting a person with a learning disability, it may be important to ascertain what their usual teeth-cleaning routine is, as they may not be able to tell you.

People with mental health problems – who are severely depressed, for example – may not view their personal hygiene as important, so both physical and psychological support could be required.

When caring for a child, encourage and assist parents or carers to be involved in hygiene care to maintain the usual routine. Supporting, educating and enabling parents or carers to continue their care within any environment is an important nursing role.

☑ Care-setting considerations

Ensure dignity is maintained, as most individuals carry out all of their hygiene practices in private.

Teeth-cleaning can be undertaken in any care setting.

☑ What to watch out for and action to take

Remember to constantly observe and assess the person's tongue and oral structures. If you observe any areas that are abnormal, you need to report this to a relevant individual and record it in the person's notes.

Teeth-cleaning assistance guidelines

Perform steps 1-7 of the Hygiene assistance guidelines (pp. 144-145)
Prepares the person and yourself to undertake the task.

Drape a towel around the person's front
Protects clothes.

 Apply a pea-sized blob of toothpaste to the toothbrush. Ask the person to open their mouth and, holding the brush at 45 degrees, use small circular motions to brush the teeth
Effectively cleans teeth.

 Brush the upper teeth first, brushing all surfaces, paying extra attention to the area where the teeth and gums meet
Particles gather between the teeth and gums.

 When you have brushed all areas, offer the person diluted mouthwash or water to rinse
Removes toothpaste and particles.

 Assist the person to look at their teeth in the mirror to ensure they approve of the result
Enables the person to present themselves in the manner they desire.

 Perform steps 8-10 of the Hygiene assistance guidelines (p. 145)
To ensure that:

- the person is safe, comfortable and receiving the appropriate care
- the results have been documented in the person's records
- the equipment is clean and in working order.

Source: Baillie et al. (2014); Lister et al. (2020); NICE (2017); NMC (2018); Price and McAlinden (2017); Steel (2017)

Trimming nails

☑ What is normal

Most patients have their own hygiene practices, which may be very different from yours, so remember to ensure you are working in partnership with your patient. Remember to constantly observe and assess the condition of the patient's nails and surrounding skin.

☑ Before you start

Remember to perform the common steps (Hygiene assistance guidelines, (pp. 144–145).

☑ Essential equipment

Scissors, nail clippers, nail file, soap/hand cleanser, bowl, warm water, towel, hand-lotion if the patient wishes.

☑ Care setting considerations

It is possible to trim a patient's nails in all settings as long as the necessary equipment is available.

☑ What to watch out for and action to take

If any areas of skin or any nails have been observed which are abnormal this must be reported to a relevant individual and recorded in the patient's notes.

Trimming nails guidelines

1 **Perform steps 1–7 of the Hygiene assistance guidelines (pp. 144–145). Offer assistance as required to prepare the patient so you are able to access the nails you are going to trim. Only uncover the area you are working on. Assist the patient to find a comfortable position**
To prepare the patient and yourself to undertake the skill.
Maintains patient dignity. If you are at the patient's bed space ensure you draw the curtains fully.

2 **Fill a bowl with fresh warm water, check the temperature carefully and if possible check that the patient is happy with the temperature. Change this water at any time if it becomes too cool or dirty**
Patient safety.
  Reduces risk of contamination.

3 Ensure the bowl and the patient are at a height at which it is comfortable for you to work, changing this throughout the procedure as necessary
Cares for your back.

4 Trimming fingernails
Soak the patient's hands in the water and gently clean around and underneath their nails if required.

5 Trimming toenails
Soak the patient's feet in the water, wash their feet and gently clean around and underneath their nails if required. Check their feet for any signs of:

- redness, warmth, soreness or pain (infection)
- numbness or tingling (neuropathy)
- dry or cracked skin
- swelling
- blisters, cuts, scratches or sores
- in-growing toenails, corns, calluses
- toenail fungus (discolouration).

If you find any of the above report it to your practice eductor or a registered nurse.
Reduces risk of contamination.

6 Assess the condition of the skin and nails and ensure any potential problems are reported.
Dry the patient's hands and nails carefully. Dry the patient's feet very carefully, especially between their toes.
To promote comfort and prevent the patient from feeling cold.

7 Trim one nail at a time. Cut the nail straight across. Do not cut down into the corners; you should still be able to see the white tip at the top edge. If after trimming any of the nails still have a rough edge wait until the nail is properly dry and then file it smooth
To ensure nails are not cut too short and are smooth so they do not catch on clothing or scratch skin.

8 Apply hand-lotion if the patient wishes
If the patient desires you can apply lotion to the top and bottom of their feet, but not between the toes.

Dispose of bowl or clean with detergent and water if reusable. Store inverted to avoid dregs of water collecting in it.

9 **Dispose of/clean any other equipment as per local policy and return any of the patient's equipment to their locker. If appropriate clean the bedside table and put any belongings you moved back in their original position. Ensure the patient can reach the nurse call bell**
Reduces risk of infection.
Maintains patient safety.

10 **Perform steps 8-10 of the Hygiene assistance guidelines (p. 145)**
To ensure that the:

- patient is safe, comfortable and receiving the appropriate care
- results have been documented in the patient's records
- equipment is clean and in working order.

Source: Baillie (2014); Dougherty et al. (2015); Glasper et al. (2010); NICE (2012a); NMC (2018); Sargeant and Chamley (2013)

Washing a patient's hair in bed

☑ What is normal

Most patients have their own hygiene practices, which may be very different from yours, so remember to ensure you are working in partnership with your patient.

Remember to constantly observe and assess the condition of the patient's hair and skin on their scalp.

☑ Before you start

Remember to perform the common steps (Hygiene assistance guidelines (pp. 144-145).

☑ Essential equipment

Bed hair-rinser, towel x3, large incontinence pads, patient's shampoo, brush and comb, bowl x2, warm water, jug, mirror and any other hair product the patient uses.

☑ **Care setting considerations**

It is possible to wash a patient's hair in bed in any setting as long as the necessary equipment is available.

☑ **What to watch out for and action to take**

If whilst washing a patient's hair any areas of skin have been observed which are abnormal this must be reported to a relevant individual and recorded in the patient's notes.

Washing a patient's hair guidelines

1 **Perform steps 1-7 of the Hygiene assistance guidelines (pp. 144-145)**
To prepare the patient and yourself to undertake the skill.

2 **Offer assistance as required to prepare the patient. Draw the curtains fully around the patient's bed space if appropriate. Clear sufficient space around the patient's bed, pull it out so you can easily access the head end, and ensure you reapply the brakes. Wrap a towel around the patient's shoulders**
Maintains patient dignity and keeps them warm.
To enable you to move freely in the bed space.
To stop them from getting wet.

3 **Make sure that the patient is comfortable whilst you are undertaking the next step, 'preparing the bed and bedspace', moving them following safe patient moving principles**
To promote patient comfort.
Preparing the bed space effectively is most important, as otherwise the procedure will not go smoothly.

4 **Lay the patient and the bed flat, so you can either fold the bed's headboard down, as some can be used as a shelf at the top of the bed, or remove it completely. If the headboard cannot be used as a shelf move the patient's bed table to this position, as this is where the bed hair-rinser will go. Position another table as close to the top of the bed as possible and place the jug and a bowl of clean warm water on this table**

Ensure that the patient is able to tolerate lying flat.
To effectively prepare the bed space.
To enable equipment to be at hand when you need it.

 Place a towel on the bed head or table and place the bed hair-rinser on top. Position the spout so it hangs over the side; place a large incontinence pad on the floor underneath this with an empty bowl on top to collect the waste water
To prevent water from escaping and wetting the floor.

 Assist or move the patient to a comfortable position where their head is laying in the bed hair-rinser
To ensure the patient is in the correct position to have their hair washed.

 Use the jug to wet the patient's hair with the warm water in the bowl. Check that the patient is happy with the temperature of the water and protect their eyes and ears. Do not hurry and be gentle
To promote patient comfort whilst washing their hair.

 Put a small amount of shampoo on the palm of your hand and rub it into the patient's hair and scalp with circular movements. Rinse the hair with warm water, repeating as often as necessary until all of the lather from the shampoo has been washed away. Repeat the shampooing and rinsing stages until the hair is clean

 Wrap a clean towel around the patient's hair and assist or move their head out of the bed hair-rinser
To remove equipment no longer required.

 Ensure the patient is in a comfortable position and ask them how they wish their hair to be styled. If local policy allows use a hairdryer to dry their hair
To promote patient comfort.

 Assist the patient to look at their hair in a mirror to ensure they approve of the result. Remove the towel from the patient's shoulders and ensure they are in a comfortable position
To ensure the patient is happy with the end result of their hair washing and drying.

12 **Dispose of bowls or clean with detergent and water if reusable. Store inverted to avoid dregs of water collecting in them. Dispose of/clean any other equipment as per local policy and return any of the patient's equipment to their locker. Clean the bedside table and put any belongings you moved back in their original position. Ensure the patient can reach the nurse call bell**
Reduces risk of infection.
  Maintains patient safety.

13 **Perform steps 8-10 of the Hygiene assistance guidelines (p. 145)**
To ensure that the:

- patient is safe, comfortable and receiving the appropriate care
- results have been documented in the patient's records
- equipment is clean and in working order.

Source: Baillie (2014); Dougherty et al. (2015); Glasper et al. (2010); NICE (2012a); NMC (2018); Sargeant and Chamley (2013)

CARE AFTER DEATH
MARIA PARRY

☑ **Before you start**

Two or more healthcare professionals should complete the care after death procedure. This personal care is the responsibility of the registered nurse/home manager, although some tasks such as property management can be delegated. Personal care, if appropriate to be completed, needs to be concluded within a 4-hour window.

☑ **Essential equipment**

Nurses must prepare the area and wear disposable aprons and gloves (Covid-19 guidelines will apply here). The dignity and privacy of the patient must always be maintained.

☑ **What to watch out for**

It is imperative that manual handling guidance is adhered to.
   Shaving can cause bruising if completed while the person is warm, so should be avoided, unless specifically requested. This may be not wished for on cultural and religious grounds.

Care after death guidelines

 As soon as possible following death, the person should be laid flat with the head supported by one pillow. Where possible straighten limbs and place the arms by the person's side

2 Completing this first part of the process will involve closing the eyes, which can require slight pressure on the eyelids, and cleaning the mouth area of any debris, placing any teeth or dentures in the patient's mouth

 3 Mechanical devices need to be removed such as intravenous infusions, syringe driver pumps and urine catheter bags. Any internal tubes such as cannulas, catheters, Hickman or central venous pressure lines may be required to be left in situ, depending on the local policy and if the death needs referral to the coroner. Local guidelines need to be checked

 4 To ensure the bladder is drained, gentle pressure is placed on the lower abdomen as bodies can excrete fluids after death; genitalia also need to be included in the bed bath, changing flannels as necessary, and wipes may be used here to assist

 5 Pads and pants can be utilised to absorb any leakage of fluid from the urethra, vagina or rectum. Cover any stomas with a clean bag

 6 Cover all wounds that have exudate with a clean absorbent dressing. Clamp any drains and cover with occlusive dressing

 7 The bed bath should be commenced as you would with an unconscious patient, starting with the face

8 The patient should be rolled abiding by manual handling techniques to fully clean the patient. Some patients will expel air or fluids that may be contained in the lungs or gastrointestinal tract, this can be a normal response to movement

9 A clean, dry sheet should be inserted under the patient, which will eventually be used to wrap the patient for transportation. The patient should be dressed, still ensuring privacy and dignity, with a hospital shroud, gown or the patient's preferred clothing. The person should not go to the mortuary naked

 10 The notification of death label is placed on the patient's chest; identification tags are also placed onto one wrist and one ankle (community and hospital)

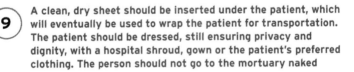

The sheet inserted under the patient is wrapped around the patient, covering the patient's face, and secured in place with tape. The feet are also covered. The second notification of death is placed on top of the sheet and secured with tape

 Covering the patient's face is necessary to avoid possible damage to the body during transfer and avoid distressing any staff

 Depending on the health board policy and infection control procedures a body bag may be used. If this is the case, the second notification of death label is placed onto the body bag, with any transportation/infection control documentation (Covid-19 will necessitate the use of a body bag)

 Once the patient has been prepared appropriately to be moved to the mortuary, the portering staff can be contacted. While the body is being removed other patients and relatives can be screened off to avoid any unnecessary distress from the ward areas

 It is important to remember that this can be a distressing experience for nurses

 Ensure mortuary staff and funeral directors are informed of any potential for profuse leakage to enable appropriate positioning of the deceased

 Avoid waterproof, strongly adhesive tape as this can be difficult to remove at the funeral directors and can leave a permanent mark

Source: Adapted from Hospice UK (2015); Jones and Parry (2019)

APPENDIX 1

COMMONLY USED MEDICATION AND SIDE EFFECTS

WENDY WRIGHT AND FIONA EVERETT

You should also check the cautions, contraindications and dose. Continue to build up your list of known medication following the information below.

Cardiovascular system		
Name	**Indications**	**Side effects**
Amlodipine	Hypertension, prophylaxis of angina	Abdominal pain, nausea, palpitations, flushing, oedema, headache, dizziness, sleep disturbances, fatigue
Aspirin	Secondary prevention of thrombotic cerebrovascular or cardiovascular disease	Bronchospasm, gastro-intestinal irritation, gastrointestinal haemorrhage
Atenolol	Hypertension, angina, arrhythmias	Gastrointestinal disturbances, bradycardia, heart failure, hypotension
Atorvastatin	Hypercholesterolemia	Myalgia, myopathy, gastro-intestinal disturbances, sleep disturbances, headache, dizziness

Cardiovascular system

Name	Indications	Side effects
Digoxin	Heart failure, supraventricular arrhythmias	Nausea, vomiting, diarrhoea, arrhythmias, dizziness, blurred vision, rash
Diltiazem	Prophylaxis and treatment of angina, hypertension	Bradycardia, palpitations, dizziness, hypotension, malaise, headache, hot flushes, oedema
Glyceryl trinitrate	Angina	Postural hypotension, tachycardia, throbbing headache, dizziness
Isosorbide mononitrate	Prophylaxis of angina, adjunct in congestive cardiac failure	Postural hypotension, tachycardia, throbbing headache, dizziness
Lisinopril	Hypertension and heart failure	Hypotension, renal impairment, persistent dry cough, rash
Nicorandil	Prophylaxis and treatment of stable angina	Nausea, vomiting, rectal bleeding, flushing, increase in heart rate, dizziness, headache
Nifedipine	Prophylaxis of angina, hypertension	Gastro-intestinal disturbances, hypotension, oedema, vasodilatation, palpitations, headache, dizziness, lethargy
Pravastatin	Hypercholesterolemia	Myalgia, myopathy, gastro-intestinal disturbances, sleep disturbances, headache, dizziness
Ramipril	Hypertension, symptomatic heart failure	Hypotension, renal impairment, persistent dry cough
Simvastatin	Hypercholesterolemia	Myalgia, myopathy, gastro-intestinal disturbances, sleep disturbances, headache, dizziness
Spironolactone	Oedema and ascities	Gastro-intestinal disturbances, malaise, confusion, drowsiness, dizziness

Central nervous system

Name	Indications	Side effects
Carbamazepine	Focal and secondary generalised tonic-clonic seizures, trigeminal neuralgia	Headache, ataxia, drowsiness, nausea, vomiting, blurred vision
Citalopram	Depressive illness, panic disorder	Nausea, vomiting, dyspepsia, abdominal pain, diarrhoea, constipation, anorexia, rash
Co-codamol	Mild to moderate pain	Nausea, vomiting, constipation, dry mouth, biliary spasm, respiratory depression, hypotension, muscle rigidity
Diazepam	Short-term use in anxiety and insomnia, adjunct in acute alcoholic withdrawal	Drowsiness and light headedness the next day, confusion, ataxia, amnesia, dependence, muscle weakness
Fluoxetine	Major depression, bulimia nervosa, obsessive compulsive disorder	Diarrhoea, dysphagia, vasodilation, hypotension, flushing, palpitations
Lorazepam	Status epilepticus, febrile convulsions	Drowsiness and light headedness the next day, confusion, ataxia, amnesia, dependence, muscle weakness
Methadone	Severe pain, cough in terminal disease, adjunct in treatment of opioid dependence	Nausea, vomiting, constipation, dry mouth, biliary spasm
Morphine sulphate	Severe pain	Nausea, vomiting, constipation, dry mouth, biliary spasm
Paracetamol	Mild to moderate pain, pyrexia	Side effects rare
Paroxetine	Major depression, obsessive-compulsive disorder, panic disorder, post-traumatic stress disorder	Nausea, vomiting, dyspepsia, abdominal pain, diarrhoea, constipation, anorexia, rash

Central nervous system

Name	Indications	Side effects
Risperidone	Schizophrenia and other psychoses	Tremor, dystonia, restlessness, sexual dysfunction, tachycardia, arrhythmias, hypotension
Sertraline	Depressive illness, obsessive-compulsive disorder, panic disorder	Nausea, vomiting, dyspepsia, abdominal pain, diarrhoea, constipation, anorexia, rash
Temazepam	Insomnia	Drowsiness and light headedness, confusion, ataxia
Tramadol	Moderate to severe pain	Nausea, vomiting, constipation, dry mouth, biliary spasm, diarrhoea, retching, fatigue
Venlafaxine	Major depression, generalised anxiety disorder	Constipation, nausea, anorexia, weight changes, vomiting, hypertension, palpitations
Zopiclone	Insomnia	Taste disturbance, nausea, vomiting, dizziness, drowsiness, dry mouth, headache

Endocrine system

Name	Indications	Side effects
Gliclazide	Used in diabetes	Gastro-intestinal disturbances
Levothyroxine	Hypothyroidism	Diarrhoea, vomiting, angina pain, arrhythmias, palpitations, tachycardia, tremor, restlessness
Metformin	Diabetes mellitus	Anorexia, nausea, vomiting, diarrhoea, abdominal pain, taste disturbance

Gastro-intestinal system

Name	Indications	Side effects
Lactulose	Constipation	Nausea, vomiting, flatulence, cramps and abdominal discomfort

Gastro-intestinal system

Name	Indications	Side effects
Lansoprazole	Gastric ulcer, eradication of Helicobacter pylori	Nausea, vomiting, abdominal pain, flatulence, diarrhoea, constipation and headache
Omeprazole	Gastric and duodenal ulcers	Gastro-intestinal disturbances, headache, agitation, impotence
Ranitidine	Benign gastric and duodenal ulceration, dyspepsia	Diarrhoea, headache, dizziness
Senna	Constipation	Abdominal cramp

Infections

Name	Indications	Side effects
Amoxicillin	Urinary tract infections, sinusitis, bronchitis	Nausea, vomiting, diarrhoea, rashes
Cefalexin	Broad-spectrum antibiotic which is used to treat septicaemia, pneumonia, meningitis, biliary-tract infections, peritonitis and urinary-tract infections	Diarrhoea, nausea and vomiting, abdominal discomfort, headache, rashes
Erythromycin	Oral infections, campylobacter enteritis, syphilis, respiratory tract infections, skin infections	Nausea, vomiting, abdominal discomfort, diarrhoea
Flucloxacillin	Otitis externa, adjunct in pneumonia, impetigo, cellulitis	Gastro-intestinal disturbances
Metronidazole	*Clostridium difficile* infections, leg ulcers and pressure sores, bacteria vaginosis, ulcerative gingivitis, oral infections	Gastro-intestinal disturbances, taste disturbances, furred tongue, oral mucositis, anorexia

Musculoskeletal and joint disease

Name	Indications	Side effects
Ibuprofen	Pain and inflammation in rheumatic disease, mild to moderate pain, migraine, dental pain	Gastro-intestinal disturbances including discomfort, nausea, diarrhoea, occasionally bleeding and ulceration

Musculoskeletal and joint disease

Name	Indications	Side effects
Naproxen	Pain and inflammation in rheumatic disease, dysmenorrhoea, acute gout	Gastro-intestinal disturbances including discomfort, nausea, diarrhoea, occasionally bleeding and ulceration

Nutrition and blood

Name	Indications	Side effects
Ferrous sulphate	Iron-deficiency anaemia	Gastro-intestinal irritation, nausea, epigastric pain, diarrhoea, constipation
Folic acid	Anaemia	Gastro-intestinal disturbances

Respiratory system

Name	Indications	Side effects
Salbutamol	Asthma, conditions associated with reversible airways obstruction	Fine tremor, nervous tension, headache, muscle cramps, palpitations

Source: www.medicinescomplete.com/mc/bnf/current

APPENDIX 2

NORMAL LABORATORY VALUES

WENDY WRIGHT AND FIONA EVERETT

Adult	Child			
Haematology:	**RBC**	**Male**	**Female**	μ/L = mm3
Red Blood Cells (RBC)	6 months	4.2-5.5	3.4-5.4 x	106 / μ/L
Men 4.5-6.5 x 1012/L	6 months-2 years	4.1-5.0	4.1-4.9 x	106/ μ/L
Women 3.9-5.6 x 1012/L	2-12 years	4.0-4.9	4.0-4.9 x	106 / μ/L
Haemoglobin (Hb) Men 135-175 g/L Women 115-155 g/L	12-18 years	42-53	40-49	
White Blood Cells (WBC)	**Hb**	**Male**	**Female**	
Men 3.7-9.5 x 109/L	Newborn	14.7-18.6	12.7-18.3g/dL	
Women 3.9-11.1 x 109/L	6 months-2 years	10.3-12.4	10.4-12.4g/dL	
	2-6 years	10.5-12.7	10.7-12.7g/dL	
	6-12 years	11.0-13.3	10.9-13.3g/dL	
	12-18 years	11.5-14.8	11.2-13.6g/dL	

Adult	Child		
Platelets Men 150-400 x 109/L Women 150-400 x 109/L	**WBC**		
	Newborn	6.8-13.3	8.0-14.3 x 103 / µml/L
	2 years	6.2-14.5	6.4-15.0 x 103 / µml/L
Coagulation/INR	6 months-2 years	6.2-14.5	6.4-15.0 x 103 / µml/L
INR range 2-3 (in some cases a range of 3-4.5 is acceptable)	2-6 years	5.3-11.5	5.3-11.5 x 103 / µml/L
Biochemistry:	**Platelets**		
	Newborn	164-351	234-346 x 103 / µl/L
Sodium 135-145 mmol/L	1-2 months	275-567	295-615 x 103 / µl/L
	2-6 months	275-566	288-598 x 103 / µl/L
Potassium 3.5-5.2 mmol/L	6 months-2 years	219-452	229-465 x 103 / µl/L
Urea 2.6-6.5 mmol/L	2-6 years	204-405	204-402 x 103 / µl/L
	6-12 years	194-364	183-369 x 103 / µl/L
	12-18 years	165-332	185-335 x 103 / µl/L
Creatinine 55-105 µmol/L	**Sodium** Newborn 133-146 mmol/L Children 135-145 mmol/L		

Adult	Child		
Calcium 2.2-2.6 mmol/L	**Potassium** Premature newborn 4.5-7.2 mmol/L Full term newborn 3.7-5.2 mmol/L Children 3.5-5.8 mmol/L		
	Urea 1-3 years 1.8-6.0 mmol/L 4-13 years 2.5-6.0 mmol/L 14-19 years 2.9-7.5 mmol/L		
C reactive protein (CRP) <10mg/L	**Creatinine**	**Male**	**Female**
	1-3 days	17.7-88.4	7.7-88.4 µmol/L
	1 year	17.7-53.0	17.7-44.2 µmol/L
	2-3 years	17.7-61.9	26.5-53.0 µmol/L
	4-7 years	17.7-70.7	7.7-61.9 µmol/L
	8-10 years	26.5-79.6	26.5-70.7 µmol/L
	11-12 years	26.5-88.4	26.5-79.6 µmol/L
	13-17 years	26.5-106.1	26.5-97.2 µmol/L
	18-20 years	44.2-115	26.5-97.2 µmol/L
Albumin 35-50g/L	**Calcium** Premature newborn (first week) 1.7-2.3 mmol/L Full term newborn (first week) 2.0-2.5 mmol/L Children 2.2-2.6 mmol/L		

Adult	Child
Bilirubin (Total)< 17 µmol/L	**Albumin**
	Newborn 2.6-3.6 g/dL
	1-3 years 3.4-4.2 g/dL
	4-6 years 3.5-5.2 g/dL
	7-9 years 3.7-5.6 g/dL
	10-19 years 3.7-5.6g/dL
	Bilirubin Neonates (total) < 10 µmol/L

APPENDIX 3

HAND-WASHING TECHNIQUE

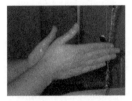

1. Wash palm to palm

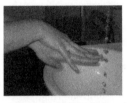

2. Rub back of both hands with interlaced fingers

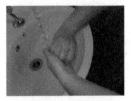

3. Rub back of fingers

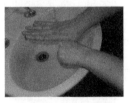

4. Wash both thumbs

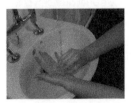

5. Rub palms with fingertips

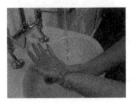

6. Wash wrists

REFERENCES

Baillie, L. (2014) *Developing Practical Adult Nursing Skills*, 4th edn. London: CRC Press.

Baillie, L., Ozenbaugh, R.L. and Pullen, T.M. (2014) *Developing Practical Nursing Skills*. London: CRC Press.

Ballentyne, M. and Ness, V. (2009) 'Eliminating', in C. Docherty and J. McCallum (eds), *Foundation Clinical Nursing Skills*. Oxford: Oxford University Press. pp. 275–307.

Best, C. and Shepherd, E. (2020) 'Accurate measurement of weight and height 1: Weighing patients'. *Nursing Times*, 116(4): 50–2.

Black, J. and Simende, A. (2020) 'Ten top tips: Assessing darkly pigmented skin', *Wounds International Journal*, 11(3): 8–11. Available at: www.woundsinternational.com/journals/issue/624/articledetails/ten-top-tips-assessing-darkly-pigmented-skin (accessed 19 March 2021).

British National Formulary (2021) *British National Formulary*, 82nd edn. London: BMJ Publishing Group Ltd and Royal Pharmaceutical Society.

Dougherty, L., Lister, S. and West-Oram, A. (2015) *The Royal Marsden Manual of Clinical Nursing Procedures*. Oxford: Wiley-Blackwell.

Glasper, A., Aylott, M. and Battrick, C. (2010) *Developing Practical Skills for Nursing Children and Young People*. London: Hodder Arnold.

Hall, C. (2018) 'Medicines administration', in C. Delves-Yates (ed.), *Essentials of Nursing Practice*, 2nd edn. London: SAGE.

Health Protection Scotland (2014) *Targeted Literature Review: What are the Key Infection Prevention and Control Recommendations to Inform a Peripheral Vascular Catheter (PVC) Maintenance Care Quality Improvement Tool?* Available at: www.hps.scot.nhs.uk/resourcedocument.aspx?id=6372 (accessed 1 May 2018).

HM Coroner (2017) *Regulation 28 Report to Prevent Future Deaths*. Available at: www.judiciary.gov.uk/wp-content/uploads/2017/06/Haughey-2017-0116.pdf (accessed 4 June 2017).

Hospice UK (2015) *Care After Death Publication Update With New Guidance for Registered Nurses on Verification of Expected Deaths*. Available at: www.hospiceuk.org/what-we-offer/publications?cat=72e54312-4ccd-608d-ad24-ff0000fd3330 (accessed 10 June 2021).

HSE (2013) *The Health and Safety (Sharp Instruments in Healthcare) Regulations 2013*. Available at: www.legislation.gov.uk/uksi/2013/645/made (accessed 25 March 2015).

Japp, A. and Robertson, C. (2018) *Macleod's Clinical Diagnosis*, 2nd edn. London: Elsevier.

Jones, B. and Parry, M. (2019) 'The rationale for making a short DVD in relation to the last offices procedure', *International Journal of Palliative Nursing*, 25(2): 91-7.

Kinoshita, K., Azuhata, T., Kawano, D. et al. (2015) 'Relationships between pre-hospital characteristics and outcome in victims of foreign body airway obstruction during meals', *Resuscitation*, 88: 63-7.

Hunter, D. (2012) 'Conditions affecting the foreskin', *Nursing Standard*, 26(37): 35-9.

Leaver, R.B. (2007) 'The evidence for urethral meatal cleansing', *Nursing Standard*, 21(41): 39-42.

Loveday, H., Wilson, J., Pratt, R., Golsorkhi, M., Tingle, A., Bak, A., Browne, J., Prieto, J. and Wilcox, M. (2013) 'EPIC 3, national evidence-based guidelines for preventing healthcare-associated infections in NHS hospitals in England', *Journal of Hospital Infection*, 86(S1): S1-S70.

Lister, S., Hofland, J. and Grafton, H. (eds) (2020) *The Royal Marsden Hospital Manual of Clinical Nursing Procedures*, 10th edn. Oxford: Wiley-Blackwell.

McCallum, L. and Higgins, D. (2012) 'Measuring body temperature', *Nursing Times*, 108(45): 20-2.

National Institute for Health and Care Excellence (NICE) (2012a) *Prevention and Control of Healthcare-Associated Infections in Primary and Community Care. Clinical Guideline 139*. London: NICE. Available at: http://guideline.nice.org.uk/CG139 (accessed 24 March 2015).

National Institute for Health and Care Excellence (NICE) (2012b) *Quality Standard for Nutrition Support in Adults*. London: NICE.

National Institute for Health and Care Excellence (NICE) (2014a) *Acutely Ill Patients in Hospital*. Available at: http://pathways.nice.org.uk/pathways/acutely-ill-patients-in-hospital (accessed 30 October 2014).

National Institute for Health and Care Excellence (NICE) (2014b) *Pressure Ulcers: Prevention and Management of Pressure Ulcers. Clinical Guideline 179*. London: NICE. Available at: www.nice.org.uk/guidance/cg179/resources/guidance-pressure-ulcers-prevention-andmanagement-of-pressure-ulcers-pdf (accessed 2 March 2015).

National Institute for Health and Clinical Excellence (NICE) (2017) *Healthcare-Associated Infections: Prevention and Control in Primary and Community Care. Clinical Guideline 139*. London: NICE. Available at: www.nice.org.uk/guidance/cg139 (accessed 10 November 2021).

National Institute for Health and Care Excellence (NICE) (2019) *Surgical Site Infections: Prevention and Treatment* [NG125]. Available at: www.nice.org.uk/guidance/ng125 (accessed 4 March 2020).

National Patient Safety Agency (NPSA) (2011) *Reducing the Harm Caused by Misplaced Nasogastric Feeding Tubes in Adults, Children and Infants*. Available at: www.nrls.npsa.nhs.uk/alerts/?entryid45=129640&q=0%C2%ACnasogastric+feeding+tubes%C2%AC (accessed 23 May 2018).

National Patient Safety Agency (NPSA) (2012) *Harm from Flushing of Nasogastric Tubes before Confirmation of Placement*. Available at: www.nrls.npsa.nhs.uk/resources/?entryid45=133441&q=0%C2%ACnasogastric+tubes%C2%AC (accessed 24 March 2015).

National Prescribing Centre (NPC) (n.d.) *A Guide to Good Practice in the Management of Controlled Drugs in Primary Care (England)*. Available at: www.npc.nhs.uk/controlled_drugs/resources/controlled_drugs_third_edition.pdf (accessed 24 March 2015).

NHS Greater Glasgow and Clyde (2017) *Standard Operating Procedure (OP): Insertion and Maintenance of Adult Indwelling Urethral Urinary Catheters*. Available at: http://live.nhsggc.org.uk/media/244826/2017-02-sop-urinary-catheters-v5-final.pdf (accessed 23 September 2020).

Nursing and Midwifery Council (NMC) (2018) *The Code: Professional Standards of Practice and Behaviour for Nurses, Midwives, and Nursing Associates*. London: Nursing and Midwifery Council.

Oxford University Hospitals NHS Trust (2016) *Oxford Pelvic Floor Service: Obstructive Defaecation*. Patient Advice and Information Leaflet on the Management of Obstructive Defaecation. Available at: www.ouh.nhs.uk/patient-guide/leaflets/files13303Polostructive.pdf (accessed 17 May 2018).

Paton, M. and Elliot, K. (2017) *Assessment of Breathing*. Elsevier Clinical Skills. Available at: www.elsevierclinicalskills.co.uk/SampleSkill/tabid/112/sid/1720/Default.aspx#&&index=7 (accessed 2 January 2021).

Price, J. and McAlinden, O. (eds) (2017) *Essentials of Nursing Children and Young People*. London: SAGE.

Public Health England (2014a) *Investigation of Faecal Specimens for Enteric Pathogens. UK Standards for Microbiology Investigations*. Bacteriology: B30 issue no. 8.1. London: Public Health England. Available at: www.gov.uk/government/uploads/system/uploads/attachment_data/file/343955/B_30i8.1.pdf (accessed 3 March 2015).

Public Health England (2014b) *Investigation of Urine: UK Standards for Microbiology Investigations*. Bacteriology: B41 issue no. 7.2. London: Public Health England. Available at: www.gov.uk/government/uploads/system/uploads/attachment_data/file/343969/B_41i7.2.pdf (accessed 3 March 2015).

Public Health England (2015) *Investigation of Throat Related Specimens*. Bacteriology, B9 Issue 9. London: Public Health England. Available at: www.gov.uk/government/uploads/system/uploads/attachment_data/file/423204/B_9i9.pdf (accessed 14 May 2021).

Public Health England (2018) *Investigation of Swabs from Skin and Superficial Soft Tissue Infections.* Bacteriology, B11 Issue 6.5. London: Public Health England. Available at: https://assets.publishing.service.gov.uk/government/uploads/system/uploads/attachment_data/file/766634/B_11i6.5.pdf (accessed 14 May 2021).

Public Health England (2019) *Investigation of Bronchoalveolar Lavage, Sputum and Associated Specimens.* Bacteriology, B57 Issue 3.5. Available at: https://assets.publishing.service.gov.uk/government/uploads/system/uploads/attachment_data/file/800451/B_57i3.5.pdf (accessed 14 May 2021).

Reilly, J., Price, L., Lang, S., Robertson, C., Cheater, F., Skinner, K. and Chow, A. (2016) 'A pragmatic randomized controlled trial of 6-step versus 3-step hand hygiene technique in acute hospital care in the United Kingdom', *Infection Control and Hospital Epidemiology,* 37: 661-6.

Resuscitation Council UK (2021) *2021 Resuscitation Guidelines.* Available at: www.resus.org.uk/library/2021-resuscitation-guidelines (accessed 27 July 2021).

Royal College of Nursing (RCN) (2011) *Nutrition Now: Enhancing Nutritional Care.* Available at: www.rcn.org.uk/professional-development/publications/pub-003284 (accessed 17 May 2018).

Royal College of Nursing (RCN) (2013) *Sharps Safety: RCN Guidance to Support the Implementation of the Health and Safety (Sharp Instruments in Healthcare Regulations) 2013.* London: RCN.

Royal College of Nursing (RCN) (2017) *Standards for the Weighing of Infants, Children and Young People in the Acute Health Care Setting.* Available at https://www.rcn.org.uk/professional-development/publications/pub-006135 (accessed 19 January 2021).

Royal College of Nursing (RCN) (2021) *Tools of the Trade.* London: RCN.

Sargeant, S. and Chamley, C. (2013) 'Oral health assessment and mouthcare for children and young people receiving palliative care', *Nursing Children and Young People,* 25(3): 30-3.

Shepherd, E. (2018) 'Injection technique 1: administering drugs via the intramuscular route', *Nursing Times,* 114(8): 23-5.

Simons, S. and Remington, R. (2013) 'The percutaneous endoscopic gastronomy tube: A nurse's guide to PEG tubes', *Medsurg Nursing,* 22(2): 77-83.

Simpson, E. (2016) 'How to manage a choking adult', *Nursing Standard,* 31(3): 42-6.

Smith, J. and Roberts, R. (2011) *Vital Signs for Nurses: An Introduction to Clinical Observations.* Oxford: Wiley-Blackwell.

Steel, B. (2017) 'Oral hygiene and mouth care for older people in acute hospitals: Part 2', *Nursing Older People,* 29(10): 20-5.

Taylor, S.J. Allan, K., McWilliam, H. and Toher, D. (2014) 'Nasogastric tube depth: The "NEX" guideline is incorrect', *British Journal of Nursing,* 23: 12.

Verma, P. (2011) *ENT Emergencies: The Management of Choking*. Available at: https://journals-sagepubcom. ergo.southwales.ac.uk/doi/full/10.1093/innovait/inq137 (accessed 30 October 2015).

Ward, D. (2017) 'Implementing infection prevention and control precautions in the community', *British Journal of Community Nursing*, 22(3): 116-18.

Westbrook, J., Woods, A., Rob, M., Dunsmuir, W. and Day, R. (2010) 'Association of interruptions with an increased risk and severity of medication administration errors', *Archives of Internal Medicine*, 170(8): 683-90.

WHO (2009) *WHO Guidelines on Hand Hygiene in Health Care*. Available at: http://whqlibdoc.who.int/publications/2009/9789241597906_eng.pdf (accessed 24 March 2014).

WHO (2014) *Giving Safe Injections: A Guide for Nurses and Others Who Give Injections*. Available at: www.who.int/occupational_health/activities/1bestprac.pdf (accessed 5 June 2014).

WHO (2020) *Hand Hygiene for All Initiative: Improving Access and Behaviour in Health Care Facilities*. Available at: www.who.int/publications/i/item/9789240011618 (accessed 19 March 2021).